CW00455763

Psychoanalytic Group Therapy

by
Karl König, M.D.
and
Wulf-Volker Lindner

translated by
Paul Foulkes, Ph.D.

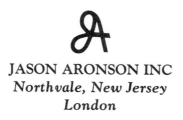

JASON ARONSON INC
Northvale, New Jersey
London

This book was set in 11 point Goudy by Lind Graphics of Upper Saddle River, New Jersey, and printed and bound by Haddon Craftsmen of Scranton, Pennsylvania.

Library of Congress Cataloging-in-Publication Data

König, Karl, 1931–
   Psychoanalytic group therapy / by Karl König and Wulf-Volker
Lindner.
      p. cm.
   Includes bibliographical references and index.
   ISBN 1-56821-119-8
   1. Group psychotherapy. 2. Social groups. I. Lindner, Wulf-
Volker. II. Title.
RC488.K68 1994
616.89'156–dc20   93-32905

Manufactured in the United States of America. Jason Aronson Inc. offers books and cassettes. For information and catalog write to Jason Aronson Inc., 230 Livingston Street, Northvale, New Jersey 07647.

THE LIBRARY OF OBJECT RELATIONS

A SERIES OF BOOKS EDITED BY
DAVID E. SCHARFF AND JILL SAVEGE SCHARFF

Object relations theories of human interaction and development provide an expanding, increasingly useful body of theory for the understanding of individual development and pathology, for generating theories of human interaction, and for offering new avenues of treatment. They apply across the realms of human experience from the internal world of the individual to the human community, and from the clinical situation to everyday life. They inform clinical technique in every format from individual psychoanalysis and psychotherapy, through group therapy, to couple and family therapy.

The Library of Object Relations aims to introduce works that approach psychodynamic theory and therapy from an object relations point of view. It includes works from established and new writers who employ diverse aspects of British, American, and international object relations theory in helping individuals, families, couples, and groups. It features books that stress integration of psychoanalytic approaches with marital and family therapy, as well as those centered on individual psychotherapy and psychoanalysis.

Refinding the Object and
  Reclaiming the Self
    David E. Scharff

Scharff Notes: A Primer of Object
  Relations Therapy
    *Jill Savege Scharff and David E.
    Scharff*

Object Relations Couple Therapy
    *David E. Scharff and Jill Savege
    Scharff*

Object Relations Family Therapy
    *David E. Scharff and Jill Savege
    Scharff*

Projective and Introjective
  Identification and the Use of the
  Therapist's Self
    Jill Savege Scharff

Foundations of Object Relations
  Family Therapy
    Jill Savege Scharff, Editor

From Inner Sources: New
  Directions in Object Relations
  Psychotherapy
    N. Gregory Hamilton, Editor

Repairing Intimacy: An Object
  Relations Approach to Couples
  Therapy
    Judith Siegel

Family and Couple Therapy
John Zinner

Close Encounters: A Relational
View of the Therapeutic Process
Robert Winer

The Autonomous Self: The Work
of John D. Sutherland
Jill Savege Scharff, Editor

Crisis at Adolescence: Object
Relations Therapy with the
Family
*Sally Box, Beta Copley,
Jeanne Magagna, and
Errica Moustaki Smilansky,
Editors*

Personal Relations Therapy:
The Collected Papers of
H. J. S. Guntrip
Jeremy Hazell, Editor

Psychoanalytic Group Therapy
*Karl Konig and Wulf-Volker
Lindner*

Psychoanalytic Therapy
Karl Konig

From Instinct to Self: Selected
Papers of W. R. D. Fairbairn,
vol. I: Clinical and Theoretical
Contributions
*David E. Scharff and
Ellinor Fairbairn Birtles, Editors*

From Instinct to Self: Selected
Papers of W. R. D. Fairbairn,
vol. II: Applications and Early
Contributions
*Ellinor Fairbairn Birtles and
David E. Scharff, Editors*

Object Relations Therapy of
Trauma
*Jill Savege Scharff and
David E. Scharff*

Object Relations Individual
Therapy
*David E. Scharff and
Jill Savege Scharff*

How to Survive as a
Psychotherapist
Nina Coltart

Reclaiming the Legacy of Erich
Fromm
*Mauricio Cortina, Daniel Burston,
and Michael Maccoby, Editors*

Contents

Part II
Special Practices

Preface

This book concerns the practice of group psychotherapy. Our hints for practice are shown to rest on theory. Our practical experience derives mainly from applying the so-called Göttingen model of group psychotherapy, which was published by Heigl-Evers and Heigl in 1973. Since then both of us have been involved in spreading the model through courses that offer personal experience, supervision, and theory. We are indebted to the participants for what we have been able to learn in working with them.

However, this is not just an account of the Göttingen model, but something of a wider scope transcending schools. We apply general concepts of psychoanalysis and social psychology to our clinical experience. The results of intensive and fruitful discussions with followers of S. H. Foulkes's school have gone into this book. Both of us have taken part in workshops of the London Group Analytic Society. In 1987 König was the first continental psychoanalytic group therapist invited to give the annual Foulkes memorial lecture.

Discussions with followers of that school were fruitful because Foulkes's network model and the Göttingen model take into account aspects from both psychoanalysis and social psychology. The two models are compatible. Readers will constantly meet basic views that mark Foulkes's concepts. We feel particularly indebted to him for the sensible division of therapeutic labor between group leader and group members. Our main interlocutors in London other than S. H. Foulkes and his wife, Elizabeth, were Malcolm Pines, Lisel Hearst, James Home, Adele Mittwoch, Herta Reik, Walter Schindler, and Hans Cohn.

Foulkes (1977) speaks of therapy *by* the group, in contrast to psychoanalysis *of* the group, as advocated by Argelander (1972), Bion (1961), and Ohlmeier (1975, 1976), as well as to psychoanalysis *in* the group, as conceived by Wolf (1971) and Sandner (1990). We think that these concepts belong to different perspectives from which one considers and uses the group process. These perspectives are not mutually exclusive. In our view, therapy by, in, and of the group may be indicated at different stages of the group process: of the group more at the beginning, by the group toward the middle and end of a group therapy. Psychoanalysis in the group is especially important if the group's conflictual situation shows clearly in a particular patient. It will then be a transition phase to therapy of and by the group.

We work in the here and now but consider it necessary to let a patient's history and relations with matters outside the group crop up. The history helps us to understand transference and resistance to it; relations with external matters tell us inter alia whether and how patients transfer insights won in the group into daily life.

We further regard a therapeutic group as an alternative system competing with other systems in which the patients live (Garland 1982). Patients try to revive the past in the group. However, the way in which they try to set up relationships confronts them with fellow patients and the therapist. One makes the origin and function of their moves intelligible to them. If their stagings are made transparent and are worked through, a new system arises for each member, which makes any new experience possible and shows its effects in other systems.

The chapters "Psychoanalytic Perception of Group Events"

and "On Ending a Group" and the section "Dealing with Dreams" in the chapter titled "Intervention," come from Wulf-Volker Lindner; "Resistance" and "Groups with Physically Ill Patients and Medical Personnel" are from both authors; the rest are from Karl König. The authors have read, discussed, corrected, and amplified each other's manuscripts, so that both can agree with the whole book.

For constructive discussions we wish to thank Mohammad Ardjomandi, Raymond Battegay, Tobias Brocher, Klaus Frank, Peter Fürstenau, Michael Hayne, Franz Heigl, Anneliese Heigl-Evers, Albrecht Hering, Reinhard Kreische, Alice Riccardi-Von Platen, Elisabeth Rohr, Raoul Schindler, Margarethe Seidl, Joseph Shaked, and Ulrich Streeck.

Some chapters of this book were originally meant for a joint publication with Franz Heigl and Anneliese Heigl-Evers. Their suggestions for the chapters on attitude to perception, resistance, working relations, preparation and initial phase of, and ending a group have been taken into account.

We also thank Elisabeth Wildhagen and Rita Rivera, who more than once typed and corrected our manuscript. Erika Dzimalle was involved in the typing of earlier publications that partly figure here. Susan Lathe, Thomas Stahlberg, and Angelika Sticheling have helped in the search for literature.

Finally, we wish to thank our wives, Gisela König and Ingrid Lindner, both of whom are also our professional colleagues, for their understanding, inspiration, and patience.

Karl König
Wulf-Volker Lindner

Overview of the Book

The introduction that follows describes how therapeutic groups differ from informal and nontherapeutic ones. In Part I, "Theoretical Foundations of Practice," we show the difference between verbal and nonverbal communication in groups. In the chapters on transference and countertransference we stress the various forms of projective identification: transference, easing of conflict, and communication. Moreover, we emphasize the account of the group as a complex system of transference triggers and the changes of this system as the group proceeds. We next define countertransference and transference of the therapist and describe their influence on various forms of therapeutic action, from indication to intervention. The therapist's neutrality is here taken as a dynamic concept, allowing some variation in his or her behavior.

In Chapter 10 we describe working relations as specifically applying to groups. We show the part of patients in the therapeutic work and the difficulties a therapist may have with giving the patients either too little or too much of the work. Resistances, insofar as they have not been dealt with before, are discussed separately in Chapter 11, underlining that we must promote not a minimum level of resistance but an optimal one, for optimal group progress.

In Chapter 12 we distinguish between descriptive and metaphorical interventions, which may consist of confrontation, clarification, or interpretation. Interpretation and answer, the latter in the sense of psychoanalytic interactional therapy of the Göttingen model, are seen as a continuum: there is no interpretation without answer from the therapist, nor answer without interpretation of relations. We describe the effects of interventions that stress the common features and those that stress differences. We also review suggestions for dealing with regression, the use of reconstructions in analytic group psychotherapy, and ways of dealing with spontaneously staged scenes induced by a patient's report. We end the chapter with a discussion of the therapist's handling of regression in psychoanalytic interactional group psychotherapy and in an analytically oriented group.

In Part II, "Special Practices," we consider silence and the speech of patient and therapist, linking both with personality structure. Here silence is not always seen as resistance. During silence, common unconscious fantasies can be built up by nonverbal signals. Chapter 15 deals with especially difficult patients who insult, castrate, manipulate, and monopolize.

Chapters 16 and 17 cover preparation and initiation of analytic group psychotherapy and ending a group, respectively. Chapters 18 and 19 apply group methods in special settings.

In Chapter 20 we distinguish group psychotherapy from group dynamics, and in Chapter 21 we examine the work of an analytic group therapist with physically ill persons and medical personnel. We end the book with a discussion of the concept of man in relation to group psychotherapy.

Introduction

Before we begin our discussion of psychoanalytic group therapy, we need to recognize the differences between a therapeutic group and an informal meeting. At a party of eight or ten, for example, conversation runs in small groups of two or three. At times all may listen to a single speaker; however, there is no rule that only one person should speak at any time.

The implicit convention, rarely spelled out, that only one person at a time should talk, in large measure determines the style of communication in a therapeutic group. This rule usually begins to function when the therapist enters the room; in some cases it starts only when all parties are present. This depends partly on the transference at work, especially as regards the therapist. However, a certain procedure may establish itself in a group and remain stable even when transference changes. The group develops a kind of tradition, such as not to start until all members have arrived. Such traditions keep possible conflict in bounds and can arise when a group meets regularly with the same or a slowly changing membership.

At a party topics vary immensely, and conversation resembles free group association (Foulkes 1977). The expert can make diagnostic inferences from this. In contrast with a therapeutic group, members do not obey the rule of free interaction (Heigl-Evers and Heigl 1968), which implies an openness not suitable for daily life outside a therapeutic group. Of course, at a party one may also speak very openly, but this tends to occur in very small groups.

Sometimes at a party one person behaves like an adviser or expert, even for psychological matters, but he is not formally appointed: asymmetry of roles is not intended. Besides, parties start and end at no precise time and the members do not just talk, they also eat and drink.

The aim of a party is different from that of a therapeutic group: those present want to enjoy themselves and exchange views; in a therapeutic group there is work to be done. Still, as in a therapeutic group, there are no verbal reports, unless formal speeches are made. If a person at a party wants to speak to the group at large, he gives a signal, for example, by tapping a glass. This conveys the request that only one person at a time is to speak. In a therapeutic group this rule is in force throughout.

We also need to consider the differences between a therapeutic group and a typical group in a work situation. Like a therapeutic group, a working group has a leader. As in the former, there usually is a rule that only one person at a time may speak. If several people talk at once, the leader decides who should proceed first. A working group usually has a well-defined task. The sequence in which the aspects of a problem are to be considered, or, in the case of several problems, which comes first, is usually fixed by a work plan or agenda. The amount of prescribed structure varies with the task and the traditions of the working group. Board meetings or general meetings of associations tend to work by an agenda previously sent to members. For urgent questions that could not be placed on the agenda, there is an item labeled "other matters." In a working group that holds brainstorming sessions, or collects ideas on a particular topic, the ideas are noted by one member or by all of them. This is fairly unstructured.

In a psychoanalytic therapeutic group there is no agenda and the topic is not prearranged. Instead, the topic is implicitly suggested, when one member talks about something that interests or preoccupies him. If enough members take up this topic, the group goes on discussing it; if not, another topic may emerge. The leader does not act in the traditional way, but usually remains in the background: unlike a working group leader, he does not explicitly open proceedings. Once the group starts, the rule of one person at a time speaking becomes operative. Since the therapeutic group leader does not lead in the traditional sense, informal group leaders arise and are supported by followers (Heigl-Evers 1978, R. Schindler 1957/1958). Often there are conflicts between subgroups or between a member and the whole group. Although the group leader neither sets the topic nor assigns speakers, the leader conveys how the group is to work by what he chooses to take up; by this the leader indicates how group events and experiences are to be regarded. Interventions consist of confrontations, clarifications, interpretations, and answers. The group leader can address individual members, subgroups, or the whole group, with everyone listening, though some members may "switch off" and not focus on the discussion. Nothing that happens in the group is exempt from the leader's comments. He can consider verbal or nonverbal interactions. If a member leaves the room, for instance, the leader may comment on why this happened just then. Hardly so in a working group.

In contrast with many working groups, analytic therapeutic groups usually do not allow smoking or drinking. In working groups smoking, drinking, and eating help to lower tension; in therapeutic groups tension is precisely not to be lowered in this way. Rather, members are to talk about inner and interpersonal tensions. As in working groups, conflicts must not become brawls. Sympathy is to be expressed verbally and not by physical touching. Communication concentrates on sight and hearing, and nonverbal aspects are confined to miming, gesture, and posture. Though most group leaders do not say so at the beginning of a session, there is generally a rule that each member stay put throughout the session. If someone is agitated or tense, he is not to resolve the tension by walking around.

Some therapists ask their patients not to meet between sessions; others allow it but expect such meetings to be discussed in the group. In a working group this would normally not be expected or allowed, since its task is not clarifying relations between members but mastering the agenda. Inner and interpersonal tensions disrupt the work. If conflicts cannot be limited through smoking, drinking, and eating, the leader tries to repel them by hints and warnings and may speak about it to individual members after the session. In an analytic group interpersonal processes are themselves the topic: they are to develop and should be clarified. In working groups running on theme-centered interaction (Cohn 1984), members discuss interpersonal tensions, but they are clarified only to the extent that they disturb the achievement of the task or theme.

Precisely because the therapeutic group leader does not lead in the traditional manner, members pay particular attention to his behavior: they seek orientation from the leader. An informal leader emerging in a group does not really occupy the leader's position. An informal leader is not the therapist; at best he can be considered a so-called assistant therapist. Interestingly, the therapist often discounts his own power and influence in an analytic group. However, by not occupying a traditional leading role and by retreating into that of a commentator, he effectively increases his influence. The group therapist thus gains a presidential role. A president who holds a largely ceremonial position, as, for example, in Germany, will be listened to, without having to prove that what he says is practicable. What the leader says, not containing direct instructions, may be put into practice by others who are politically responsible.

Such a position may be filled with varying skill and competence. A therapist who talks nonsense will soon lose any authority. If he holds back in his comments, even when asked for more direction, members will assume that he is competent, but not explicit because he thinks it inappropriate. Along with the above conscious processes there are effects of unconscious fantasies. The transference of parent figures can increase the therapist's authority, but also diminish it if the parents had little authority. A patient who experiences the therapist as incompetent may be told that this view is an imputation based on experiences with a parent figure. Of course, the therapist may actually be incompetent, but it is more likely that the suspicion derives from transference.

A truly incompetent psychotherapist will be exposed in time. Sooner or later, members will find out that he fails to understand them; they will lose interest and the group will disintegrate, for what holds them lies largely in the therapist's conveying understanding. The hope that he might be competent after all may maintain the group longer than is warranted. The leader of a working group, on the other hand, shows his competence more directly. Members of such a group mostly share with the leader a measure of specialized knowledge, which enables them to assess his work soon. In a therapy group not consisting of therapists, members usually lack such knowledge: they give the therapist provisional trust until they are convinced of his competence or incompetence.

In a therapeutic group, a member's task demands certain abilities. They relate partly to contents opposed to what is relevant in a working group. Being able to allow weaknesses, to admit a need for help and to accept it, is just as important in a patient as the ability to reflect on experience and to draw consequences from it.

Just as in a therapeutic group, the working group leader's function is to coordinate the group events. Although he usually is particularly competent in his field, he may lead the group but not enter the discussion; this may arouse doubts as to his competence, just as in a therapeutic group, when the leader's competence is not evident from his way of leading. However, the leader of a working group may take part in the discussion, assessing and arranging, so that his competence or lack of it becomes quickly obvious. Regarding his function of manifest leader, members of a working group must not try to emulate him in every way, because this runs counter to the division of labor, but they may do so as regards assessing, clarifying, and arranging: any member may arrange, summarize, and assess part of a debate. Likewise, in a therapeutic group a member may interpret; as in a working group, the leader will not always regard this as an attack on his rights, nor, if the intent is aggressive, invariably take this up.

Generally, the patient should not regard the therapist as a model of transparence or personal openness, for he offers relatively little in this way. Not so for the psychoanalytic interactional method of the Göttingen model, in which a therapist should be an example of openness. He does indeed differ from his patients in that he is selectively open in the service of the patients, whereas their openness is less selective and ministers mainly to their own therapy.

The leader of a working group, too, may offer private news, mostly in the way of small talk, to create a more personal atmosphere and loosen the run of the session; members may see this as a signal for adding something personal. The leader's task is then to prevent such discussion to predominate at the expense of the work at hand. In an analytic group carefree small talk for loosening the atmosphere is of limited use, because everything that is said may be interpreted. The therapist must avoid provoking in patients the feeling that anything said will be at once examined, illuminated, and investigated. Nevertheless, he always may do so. Small talk in a therapeutic group may be useful for establishing contact, in which case it only seems to impede the group process. A mountain is often climbed more quickly by a zigzag path than along the steepest ascent. People under strong pressure from the superego or ego ideal do not want to waste their time with small talk, but get straight to the point, to deep issues. Such behavior may be motivated by ambition, based on the need for phallic competition. Since small talk resembles free association, it is often shunned by people who are afraid to give themselves away unwittingly. Just as in a working group, it is important in therapy to be more concrete or more abstract, as the topic may demand. In a working group, general talk may hide problems: the leader asks for numbers or concrete qualitative accounts; in a therapeutic group, for feelings and accounts of concrete events. As in a working group, the therapeutic group leader can use metaphors to give brief and memorable expression to something. Although metaphors may give a clear picture of vague feelings, however, the leader must be careful not to stop at the metaphoric stage. If, for example, someone in the group says therapy feels like being "in Abraham's bosom" (see Heigl-Evers and Heigl 1977), it is important to find out whether this means the whole group or the therapist, and to what features of either the feeling of shelter or security are attached.

In working groups it will be rarer that one metaphor will be answered with another. In therapeutic groups a metaphor is often used over a long period: the group fantasizes at the metaphoric level and only later finds its way back to description, unless the metaphors are at once so obvious that everyone can translate them.

A further difference between a therapeutic and a working group is that in the latter the leader may confront a member's behavior only when it goes against generally recognized conventions, for example, interrupting a speaker or not respecting the leader's role in calling on members to speak. In contrast, the leader of a therapeutic group may question behavior that is quite within the bounds of conventions. Indeed, some conventions of daily life are suspended in therapeutic groups, particularly as regards openness of messages.

Part I

Theoretical Foundations of Practice

Chapter 1

Preliminary Remarks on the Göttingen Model of Psychoanalytic Group Therapy

This summary account is aimed at group therapists already practicing, but with a different model, for example, that of Foulkes. A beginner should read this chapter only after working through the rest of this book. He will then gain a summary overview concerning some theoretical aspects.

For different diagnoses, our model offers different group procedures. In other models, group therapeutic technique is adapted to different diagnoses by changing variables, such as

- the therapist's transparence, as regards his current psychic processes and his own life story.
- the therapist's mode of expression, which may be either more metaphorical or more descriptive.
- the structuring aspect of therapeutic action. This relates to hints given in preliminary talks and in the course of the group, when the therapist acts more or less directively regarding the behavior that he expects from group members. More than any member, he shapes the therapeutic group process by his way of acting and the extent of his frankness.
- the division of therapeutic labor between therapist and patients. Foulkes (1977), for example, wants to leave much of the work to the patients.
- the object of perception by the therapist. From the many group phenomena he selects those indicated by his theoretical concepts directing his perception. Thus he may concentrate on the group as a whole or give more attention to relations between members.
- the mode of cognitive working through the phenomena the therapist observes in the group.
- the choice of certain aspects and portions of hypothetical constructs. Different ones will be important depending on the group's composition.
- factors of the setting, such as frequency of sessions and, more rarely in outpatient than in clinical practice, their length.

The list no doubt could be continued. Some of these variants are called in psychoanalytic jargon parameters if they vary beyond a certain range (unlike Eissler 1953, who defined the term qualitatively). Even if the therapist does not mean to adapt his behavior to the patients he is treating, he does it to some extent automatically if he has empathy. His transferences and countertransferences, the makeup of his personality, his present object relations and variations in his current form, for example, through illness, can change his behavior. This, in turn, produces changes in the therapeutic process. Of these, the extent of regression is particularly important, because regression gives access to deep-lying conflicts while making demands on the ego's strength, if the regression is to be of therapeutic use and remain under control.

In the Göttingen model certain ways of behaving in the therapist are varied as to concept. Then the therapeutic process unfolds in ways appropriate to certain categories of patients. Moreover, its use by therapist and members will favor certain aspects particularly important for that category. Thus if the therapist behaves in ways promoting regression, the therapeutic process may unfold at deeper levels of regression. Basic conflicts come to the surface, manifesting themselves between members and allowing work to be done at that level. Changes of relations within the group influence the way members represent objects internally, in the sense of correction by experiences in a sequence of bringing out and reabsorbing. Thus far what happens in analytic groups corresponds to events in individual analysis. However, the group offers more scope for transference and externalizing of parts of the self onto the whole group, subgroups, individual members, or onto the therapist. In analytic group psychotherapy of the Göttingen model, this can happen on different levels of regression.

If the therapist behaves in a way that does not greatly further regression (for example, if he attends to differences between group members more than to common features, which lowers the group's power to promote regression), the group process may unfold with less regression. Work then concentrates on derived conflicts (Gill 1954), as presented in patient behavior based on character and nonregressive transferences. In Göttingen terms, this form of group therapy is called analytically oriented.

In psychoanalytic interactional therapy in the Göttingen model one does without the direct involvement of unconscious parts of conflicts, because the ego of patients to whom the procedure is applied is in any case overburdened by manifest conflicts and additional revelation of unconscious parts, though perhaps affording relief in the long run, would produce anxieties burdening the ego beyond what it can now bear. If connections are made, they relate to what the patient is conscious of. The therapist indirectly questions pathological forms of relation, by becoming available as a transparent partner and offering relations that differ from the patient's pathological relations to objects. More than in the two other procedures he helps the patient in naming and distinguishing feelings and supplying other auxiliary ego functions, while confronting the patient with the difficulties in perceiving the inner and outer world and in digesting these perceptions. Patients with a disturbed ego structure in many ways resemble those of more mature structure in a state of regression, so that they experience and behave in regressive analogy.

In the Göttingen model, analytic group psychotherapy is the dominant procedure from which analytically oriented group theory is detached, with the therapist trying to concentrate the group process onto a certain level of regression. Psychoanalytic interactional group therapy in the Göttingen model differs more strongly from mainly interpreting forms (analytic and analytically oriented): the therapist takes diagnostic account of unconscious conflicts but acts mainly on how they affect the ego. As to openness, he behaves like a patient in an analytic group, but selectively and only in the service of his therapeutic task and not for the sake of getting things off his chest or furthering his own personal development. He might indeed benefit himself, since we all develop in our therapies, but this should be a side effect and not the main motive, as is desired for patients.

In conveying the Göttingen model, the three procedures are presented in pure form, for practical and didactic reasons. However, one can combine them, or take particular aspects of therapist behavior in the model's different forms, to adapt therapeutic action to the needs of the patients concerned.

Chapter 2

Psychoanalytic Perception of Group Events

Analysts are used to concentrating heavily on the spoken word. Other things they observe in a way that Reik (1948) denoted as "listening with a third ear." With the third ear the analyst listens to things conveyed below the manifest surface of what is said. Psychoanalysts attend to mime and gesture of patients and observe body reactions that accompany feelings. In the setting of classical individual analysis visual contact is minimal: the patient does not see the analyst and the analyst sees little of the patient. By contrast, in any group therapy people sit face to face, which enhances visual perception. The psychoanalytic approach further includes introspective observation and the use of countertransference feelings and fantasies.

An example: At the first session after a forced break due to illness of the analyst, a patient begins by speaking of the analyst's telephone call canceling a session; the patient remembers that he had twice said "get well soon," which was perhaps a little excessive.

While listening to the patient, the analyst remembers the studious stress of the second wish, and he imagines slips such as the following: someone wants to drink to another's health but says "I want to sink your health." The analyst's ideas and observations as well as his countertransference to the excessive second wish and the attendant ideas related to aggression point to a latent impulse in the patient. Was the patient disappointed because of the canceled session and did he thus mean to wish the analyst something evil? In a group the analyst must attend to more phenomena than in individual analysis. He must expect that inner personal conflicts will be staged in a multipersonal fabric and up to a point enter into this (e.g., Lindner 1988). Here he is less protected than in individual analysis.

Because a group confronts the analyst with the phenomenon of multipersonal relations, he must school his power of observation to oscillate between the group as a whole and its individual members, between countertransference feelings and the attendant attitudes that he perceives by introspection. As in individual analysis, he must combine two attitudes to perception: those directed outward and inward, respectively. As regards observation, he will tend more than in individual analysis to go beyond hearing and include the visual (mime, gesture, bodily stance). He must watch the varied and complex transference triggers existing in a group (König 1976). All this makes psychoanalytic work in a group more difficult.

A beginner in group psychotherapy often tends to cling to the manifest perceptions by sound or sight and their many details. He thus protects himself against entering into phenomena of the group as a whole, which he should nevertheless take into account even when his interventions are directed to individual members. He shields himself from his own feelings and notions provoked by a group as a whole, and from the regression it may set off. In individual analysis interpersonal stagings of a patient's inner conflicts show themselves mainly in his ideas and experience and the responding feelings and ideas of the analyst, since here the visual is limited, while in groups mime and gesture have a more important role. This equally concerns the interactional part of projective identification. Since in a group more people are physically present than in individual analysis, a staging of inner conflicts can embrace more aspects at once, which makes it rather more complex than in a one-on-one relation.

Not only tyros, but even experienced analytic group psychotherapists feel taxed by the complexity of group events and the greater pull of regression. Every psychoanalyst relies on theories, even if he cannot formulate them explicitly. He always uses at least implicit basic assumptions or concepts, which shape his perceptions and help him to interpret what he observes in his patients and in his own reactions.

What seems paradoxical in the psychoanalytic approach to observation in the process of analyzing consists in trying to be as detached as possible with regard to one's own theoretical presuppositions, which indeed can never be quite achieved, but attending to a therapeutic process while consciously applying theory. The paradox dissolves if we assume that the therapist oscillates between different approaches to perception and modes of digesting what he perceives.

The gradual process of complex and many-layered events in a group acquiring shape for the therapist often begins by association with ideas. Usually such acquisitions are tested later by rational argument and thereby set into new connections with the manifest verbal contents (Argelander 1979; see also Heigl 1969).

Let us now represent one and the same sequence from a group session under different aspects, beginning with a simple account to be followed by others that are more refined and theory-based. First consider an examination of surface and latency. The former includes conscious comments of members, the latter conscious and preconscious inner and interactional processes.

An analytic group of eight patients, four men and four women, begins its first session. The therapist has had a preliminary talk with each of them alone. There has been no prior contact between members. Now they sit together for the first time and remain silent for a while. Then one of them begins to speak: "Surely we can say anything here. Why is nobody talking about himself?" Nobody replies to this in words (Lindner 1976).

The therapist notices that the members look down. She has an idea: the members look to the center of the circle as if they have come to school without any homework, as if hoping that the teacher will not see them or call on them. The therapist herself feels oppressed. After the one member's invitation to the others to speak (implicit in the question why, given the freedom to say anything, nobody spoke about himself), the therapist thinks that members are trying to look for somebody to start. Other interpretations are also possible; for example, a member who emphasizes the complete freedom, which exaggerates the rule of free interaction (Heigl-Evers and Heigl 1968), may wish to ridicule the rule by taking it to absurd lengths.

If we connect the mode of perception directed to the phenomena with the therapist's perception of her own feelings and ideas, we can make conjectures about unconscious conflicts in the group. For example, some members may externalize a strict and demanding superego, though it is not yet obvious toward whom: it may be the therapist, or the group as a whole as an object, or for a start the initiator of the session who seems to appoint himself as representative of the therapist's demand. This lies already on a metapsychological level. The patient who has spoken, the group as a whole, or the therapist is perhaps experienced as potentially meting out punishment for weakness or mistakes. The therapist reacts by feeling oppressed. This account of the sequence, distinguishing surface and underlying features, is still rather simple. If one considers the session described, the aspect of norms, formations of psychosocial compromises, and externalizing of superego structures, one can suppose that the initiator sees the rule of free expression on the basis of his own superego problems in a magnified form. Thus he advances the norm: "Here one may speak; therefore, here one must speak, and openly."

Since he merely invites others to speak about themselves but does not do so himself, he advances the implicit norm: "We should adopt this rule." Not everyone who adopts this rule must obey it; the speaker might simply urge others to follow it. In the therapist's conjectured "looking for" there might be a beginning of a psychosocial compromise of taking turns: in every session one member should offer himself as the patient, while the others apply therapy to him. In this way nothing unexpected can happen in the session; every member knows the role he occupies, without danger of unwittingly showing facets of his character that he would rather not show.

Chapter 3

When the Therapist Fails
to Understand the Group

Some therapists demand that they always understand a group process that is many-layered (they always are) in every domain and dimension. Naturally, this is impossible. The therapist should start diagnosis from the surface, proceeding to such depth as he can at the time, while observing, introspecting, and remembering events that relate to the group's history and similar situations in other groups.

Schizoid therapists often see the surface less well than the depths. They rely on their countertransference reactions unexamined as to their origin and infer impressive conclusions. Because they attend inadequately to the surface, they find it hard to dose and time their interventions, which they often fail to formulate in an assimilable form. Certain aspects of a group process corresponding to their inner world of ego and objects they grasp by projection as though intuitively, but overlook phenomena and processes that do not fit the projections of their inner world.

Analogies must be sought at various levels of abstraction. At a high level one can draw very general inferences, but these are not specific enough; at a medium level one may find therapeutically relevant structures; at a low level one may see differences more clearly than common features, and may thus overlook relevant analogies.

Schizoid therapists move too much at very abstract levels, compulsive ones too much at rather less abstract levels, attending to differences more than to common features (König 1991b).

A seminar group spoke about the difficulties of a foreign member (who happened to be absent) in finding his way about in Germany. These difficulties matched those of other members, which they had learned to bring in from individual analysis to the new field of group therapy while learning and practicing the neccessary changes in therapeutic behavior.

On a level of general abstraction one might here say that the members speak about another's difficulties while having their own. On a medium level it becomes clear what these difficulties resemble. On a low level the common feature might not be noticed, since the problems of a foreigner coming to Germany are different from those of an individual therapist when learning group therapy.

Therapists with a strong compulsive need for control or with high narcissistic demands feel a particularly strong need to understand everything immediately. Sometimes a certain perfectionism shows itself in interventions that are very carefully stated and to the point, so that members neither need, nor feel free, to adapt an intervention to their own needs.

Some therapists shrink from letting a group notice that they do not fully understand. When we fail to grasp the sound of a word or sentence, we almost always ask. What is hard to pronounce is often imprecisely articulated but usually relevant. Likewise, asking is indicated when the therapist fails to grasp the surface of group discussion.

A therapist did not understand what members were discussing. He said so and was told that a member was pregnant. She had told the others in the therapist's absence before the session began. Now the therapist understood what the members had been saying.

If the therapist admits that he cannot yet see what the group is going on about, this usually causes less anxiety than might be expected. Rather, it tends to inspire members to reflect for themselves and tell the therapist what they have understood. Contrary to advice that Greenson (1967) has given for individual analysis, we recommend that in group therapy one should not wait for the end of a session before saying that one had not understood what was being said. Greenson's advice was meant for analysis four or five times a week. If a patient knows that he will return the next day, he will be less worried that the therapist did not grasp what was going on than he would if he were not going to see the group and therapist again for a week or a few days (in a twice weekly group). We recommend that failure to understand should be mentioned at a time when members are still talking about the matter in question so that they can be induced to clarify it. We are constantly amazed at what a group is able to perform in such cases, often indeed more than the therapist on whom the group had earlier relied too much. Here we can speak of a performative advantage of the group (Hofstätter 1971).

On the other hand, a therapist should not be satisfied with simply having failed to understand something and then finding out through the group. He should reflect on why he had failed, whether perhaps this is habitual and requires self-analysis or supervision. Just as the group should not rely too much on the therapist, so the therapist should not rely too much on the group. If in groups he has a habitual problem in perceiving or assessment, he cannot count on members being always able to help him. It may be that his blind spots coincide with those of the members, or that a therapist without such blind spots can still reach a prompter result and a more effective intervention.

Chapter 4

Verbal and Nonverbal Communication

Feelings can be experienced or repressed (isolating content from emotion). If one prevents certain ideas from becoming conscious the corresponding feelings will then not arise. Conversely, feelings may become conscious without ideas, such as fear in the case of phobia. Feelings generate impulses to action, the various ego functions contributing to plans of action.

In psychoanalytic therapies a part of possible action is excluded by agreement: one speaks but does not act in other ways. This facilitates the emergence of instinctive fantasies and the rise of corresponding plans for action, because their conversion into anxiety-provoking action will be prevented (König 1991b).

In group procedures of humanist psychology that allow bodily touching, there are limits. For example, nobody must be injured. In some cases certain bodily regions are excluded. However, in analytic procedures infantile fantasies may arise in a regression promoted or induced by the setting. Here it is vital that desires that provoke fear are not converted into action within the setting, because the fears accompanying the desires can be extreme and archaic, like the impulses to act. Other members must be protected from actions that arise from such impulses.

Thus abstinence in an analytic setting has a facilitating character. While admitting action in nonanalytic groups leads to ritual forms of social intercourse, facilitating the rise of certain fantasies and impulses or plans for action, but excluding other feelings, impulses, and plans of action, the convention of psychoanalytic nonaction except on the level of speech, mime, and gesture enables one to make conscious a greater variety of features.

To experience feelings and to show them are two different matters (König 1991a). What you experience you need not always display, and if you show it too clearly you do not always experience it as intensely. If you ask a demonstrative person whether he really has this experience, it can happen that he hesitates and replies "not quite." In the course of their development, such persons have come across others who greatly valued and rewarded lively mime and gesture, so they have learned to "supply" expression of feeling. The hysterically disposed tend to do this.

In the 1970s one constantly observed that members who best met expectations of self-awareness groups, workshops, group-dynamic sessions, and patient groups were those who showed frequent and intense feelings in the group. However, many patients are weak in decoding mimic expression. Such members may demand of others that they express their feelings more intensely. They behave like people hard of hearing who imagine their interlocutors speak softly when in fact using normal volume. A therapist who in his groups favors the rule that feelings should be expressed with extreme clarity may thereby prevent a weakness in decoding from being discovered, faced, and worked on. Since feelings may be expressed by the content of what is said and by the nonverbal part of statements like voice and volume, as well as mime, gesture, and posture, emotions and moods are often simultaneously conveyed by different channels. These last may issue contrary signals, as when someone says something aggressive while smiling in order to attenuate its impact. The smile may be deliberate or may unconsciously express a positive attitude toward the person who is being criticized. However, it may also signal an unconscious sadistic impulse hiding behind a seemingly objective criticism, or simply an ambivalent attitude toward the interlocutor.

Those whose development is stuck at the preambivalent stage will see such signals as confusing and perceive them as a double bind (Sluzki and Ransom 1976). This seems to happen more often than a genuine double bind, which arises only when its creator has an active ego-split defense mechanism, with different contradictory ego states determining messages conveyed by different channels. True double binds are thus rare, while misunderstanding of ambivalence as double bind is frequent (König and Kreische 1991).

In the early days of group therapy in Germany many therapists not only demanded very clear expression of feelings, but also viewed conflicting signals via several senses (such as smiling while criticizing) simply as resistance to clearly conveying what is being said. Today we take a subtler view.

Not only feelings are expressed and conveyed nonverbally. The interactional part of projective identification in its three forms (transference, release from inner conflict, and communication; see König 1991b) uses nonverbal signals of which the user is, as a rule, not aware that he emits them. They might be simple mime or gestures, or complex actions that often include a verbal side, for example, in seductive behavior aiming at making the other into a good object extending sympathy. Likewise, provocations that lead another to behave like a bad object can be primitive or complex, crude or subtle. Through such signals earlier sets of relations can be restaged in the present, as in the case of the interactional part of transferential projective identification. In the case of release from conflict, parts of the self or the object in conflict with it are actualized in the interpersonal field. In communicative projective identification likenesses in experience are created, which in the case of schizoid persons make communication easier or indeed possible.

In groups, nonverbal communication has further functions. This has been studied in the Department of Clinical Group Psychotherapy at Göttingen University by Gerlinde Herdieckerhoff (1989), whose account will be followed in the next section.

While in therapeutic groups one usually follows the implicit rule that only one person at a time should speak, others may simultaneously communicate nonverbally, showing their interest, some other emotion, or boredom. One who no longer wishes to listen can show this nonverbally. Herdieckerhoff gives an example: the person suddenly sits up rigidly, raises his eyes, and groans. If a member is supported in what he says, this often shows by the adopting of suitable postures (Scheflen 1964). Members in mutual accord occasionally move almost together: if one person changes his posture, another will soon do the same. Scheflen pointed out that members who aim at harmony tend, under tension between subgroups, to set half their bodies into the posture of one subgroup and the other half into that of the other subgroup. Scheflen held that a basic agreement between people who are thrashing out a disagreement can be expressed by the parties adopting the same posture nevertheless, but an outsider can mark himself as such, as Herdieckerhoff emphasizes, by adopting a posture different from that of all the others.

Coalitions between members can be contracted nonverbally. If, for example, someone shows lack of interest, as in the previous example, he can be supported by nodding or perhaps imitating his eye movement, to signal agreement with him.

Moods, too, can be conveyed nonverbally. On videotapes of group sessions, Herdieckerhoff observed that aggressive verbal statements were preceded by motor unrest that seemed to transfer itself from member to member. Depressive moods as well as aggressive ones may be conveyed nonverbally. Thus on another group videotape Herdieckerhoff noted that a change of mood toward depression announced itself even before the session began by some members sitting bent over, their shoulders drooping, though the general tone seemed still to be cheerful. Such signals are on the subtle side; others are more distinct and often become very effective, as, for example, weeping, which is rarely ignored.

All nonverbal signals so far described can give hints to the therapist. He can recognize what member may be expected to remain silent, who will not speak but wants to listen, which may be expressed by a relaxed way of leaning back, and who may be expected to speak. Potential speakers often adopt a tenser posture, make more eye contact, align their feet as if about to rise, and exhibit other introductory gestures (Kendon 1977). Herdieckerhoff points out that nonverbal communication can produce a consensus on who is to start talking, just as this is sometimes done verbally. As we have personally observed, members who wish to discuss a problem where they expect help from the therapist often seat themselves opposite the latter, as they do when preparing a discussion with him. If the interlocutor is to be a member, they sit opposite that member. Those who are highly ambivalent toward the therapist often seem to sit to his left; those whose intense relation to him is positive will more likely sit near him on the right (confirming observations by Frank 1986). This can be observed above all when the therapist's seat is fixed. If seats near him at first remain empty and are taken only by those who arrive last, this often shows that fear or aggressiveness strongly determines relations to the therapist. However, a group may leave these places free for members who had them before or seem to have some right to them.

Nonverbal behavior can be a strong trigger of transference, but the fact that transference is developing can itself be nonverbally expressed. Herdieckerhoff describes how a member who was weak in standing his ground vis-à-vis his constantly nagging mother began by expressing the corresponding transference by hostile nonverbal behavior when a new female member of similar behavior attended for the first time. In the sequel he attacked her strongly. Here nonverbal behavior precedes and announces equivalent verbal behavior.

Nonverbal communication can convey complex contents when unconscious fantasies become conscious. This leads to a group's developing a shared unconscious fantasy without it being mentioned. The result arises not only by all members being exposed to the same transference trigger, but also by nonverbal communication in reacting to that trigger. Unconscious fantasies can thus convey themselves to a supervision group. One of us (König), together with a supervision group, observed a session for 45 minutes, in which all patients and the therapist were silent (not as a rule recommended behavior for a therapist). In the discussion that followed, views on the fantasies in the supervision group were exchanged and a shared unconscious one emerged that was directly linked with group events of the preceding session, which rather perplexed the therapist who knew about them. A young psychologist, who had started training at a hospital where the group was taking place, became quite anxious, because she developed the fantasy that psychoanalysts can look into people. Directly confronting nonverbal behavior in a group needs much tact and a sure touch for timing. Beginners should be careful here. The easiest is to deal with nonverbal behavior that everyone knows communicates, as, for instance, mime and gesture of arms. That one can express something by one's legs is less well known. Therefore, and also because leg position is often linked with sexuality, we recommend caution in dealing with what is thus expressed. Members who are confronted about their leg posture can feel much more strongly exposed and ashamed than those who are addressed about their arm movements. If nonverbal behavior is brought up too often, it may become overcontrolled or, especially with hysterical cases, lead to excessive performance of it. However, tackling nonverbal behavior, perhaps with confirmation by other members, can convince the performer and even get him moving.

When patients address the nonverbal behavior of another patient, they naturally do not observe the therapeutic caveats that a therapist would adopt. It may then be necessary to weaken patients' remarks on nonverbal behavior of other members or even to query them, as, for instance, one often has to when there is a discrepancy between speech and attendant behavior. If members are weak in decoding for tone, mime, and gesture, as often happens in schizoid, narcissistic, compulsive, and hysterical patients, who then urge other members to express their feelings more clearly, the therapist can say that he himself perceives these feelings and ask whether the problem is not rather one for those who urge for clearer expression. That, of course, is an intervention requiring much tact and caution.

Chapter 5

General Points on Transference and Projective Identification

Transference occurs everywhere. We all transfer earlier experiences to present events. Previous experiences with others shape our expectations, feelings, and behavior toward people we meet now. Those whom we have known before are present as memory traces that contain their qualities and the way we related to them. These traces are "inner object representations," object meaning person. Of people we come to know now we form new representations. Since we perceive people we come to know now similarly to those we already know, new object representations usually resemble older ones. As we become more closely acquainted with new people, we perceive more of their reality and the new object representations come to differ increasingly from older ones that determined how we perceived such new people.

This act of distinguishing is indeed slowed down or prevented, when we influence the new people, by the interactional part of transference (without generally noticing it) in often subtle and obscure ways (Sandler 1976), so as to make them more like people we have known in the past. As Bertolt Brecht put it, the individual forms a picture of the other and tries to make him resemble it.

The less we learn of new acquaintances, the more scope remains for fantasies and the less we need to activate the interactional part of transference to assimilate the new people to those we knew before. Thus the therapist's abstinence creates scope for fantasy.

The motive for assimilating new people to those we knew earlier is the wish for familiarity (König 1982), which also makes us feel safe, as Sandler (1960) pointed out. At the same time, we have a desire for coming to know new facts and people. This may even lead us to attend less intensely to the familiar if we regard it as less interesting; just as conversely the desire for the familiar may lead us to perceive the familiar more strongly than what is novel. Whether we wish to see more of the one than the other depends on how mature or archaic is our inner picture of the alien (Erdheim 1988). It also depends on age: the young are keener on novelty than the old (Bischof 1985). The tasks of detachment and individuation, for example, cause an adolescent to seek new models or to notice preferentially those aspects of people that distinguish newly met objects from familiar ones. However, adolescents do not always escape the basic principle that earlier experiences are transferred to new ones.

To which inner objects we assign familiar qualities depends on basic resemblances. These may consist of a person being of the same sex as an inner object; a man may remind us of our father, particularly of the strong father if the man meets us as one in authority. Not only looks but also behavior and social position of a man may act as a trigger of transference. A newly met woman, too, may remind us of our father, if she is in a position of authority and the father had such a position in the family, but the mother did not have an authoritarian position or had less of one. Other important reference figures in the primary family, such as grandparents, uncles or aunts, and siblings, are inner objects. In sum we may say that those objects that come from the primary family or its environment have the greatest influence on our later relations, since a child is more malleable than an adult. In its first five years a child interacts most often with these objects and depends on them most strongly.

Inner object representations such as those of father or mother consist of several layers. At the core is father or mother as the small child has perceived them; from the center outward the layers are arranged in chronological order. In regression earlier layers reach the surface and layers further out melt away. Regression arises when people feel anxious or helpless, but also when they enter relations with objects that in their qualities remind them of important reference figures of childhood. Our ego then approaches the conditions of that time, in ways of experiencing relations, fears, and impulses to action. Similarities of persons in the field of our outer relations with object representations of our inner world are "transference triggers" (König 1976), that is, qualities and ways of behaving that resemble those of inner object representations.

Chapter 6

Transference in Groups

Not only an individual may remind us of earlier reference persons, but a group can be experienced as a global object, which is bigger and more powerful than an individual member. At the same time the latter is part of this global object, just as in the earlier mother–child relation in which the child does not yet experience himself as separate from the mother.

A group as global object acts as a strong transference trigger for early mother-objects. Members experience the group as global object mainly at the beginning of a group therapy, when they are as yet little acquainted with one another. With growing information in the course of the group process the unknown and in some ways indistinct global object gives way to the individual members and multipersonal transferences come to the fore. A group offers transference triggers for dyadic and multipersonal relations.

Dyadic relations can exist between one person and the group or a subgroup, such as member and therapist, member and group including the therapist, or member and member. In this last case, the one who seeks the relation blots out the unwanted members. Thus it may happen that a member seems to talk to the therapist only. Or he may talk into the group without addressing anyone in particular, whether member or therapist, as nonverbal behavior shows. Foulkes (1977, 1990a,b) saw the group as a maternal global object and at the same time as a network for communication between members: they are the nodes of the net.

Desires for familiarity, for new perceptions, for satisfying instinctual needs with familiar or unknown objects, and members' needs for protection, variously weighted, all enter the "formation of psycho-social compromise" (Brocher 1967, Heigl-Evers and Heigl 1979, König 1982, Mentzos 1976). In general terms, these can be viewed as compromises between impulse and defense. Such formations are usually unstable, because they can never satisfy the needs of all members in equal measure. Moreover, the therapist can mention, clarify, and interpret them as resistances. Here we must not exceed the limit of the patient's tolerance, for this may weaken the ego, raise feelings of anxiety, guilt, and shame, and past that limit strengthen neurotic symptoms. Often, moreover, a new and less tractable form of resistance will then replace the old one; for example, silence takes over from intellectualizing. The interactional part of transference leads to restagings of earlier constellations in the family, with members viewed in different roles in turn: siblings, parents, grandparents, and the like.

In groups, this part of transference (along with transference itself one might call it "transferential projective identification") often externalizes and stages objects or ego portions to ease conflict. One's own instinctual desires with their corresponding portions of the self are projected onto other members and provoked in them in a way that influences the others to confirm by their behavior what is expected, as in the interactional part of transference. We then have not only transference onto the other but projection into the other, who then behaves as if he actually contained these portions of the self. The motive for such behavior is precisely inner easing of conflict: what one rejects in oneself is easier to fight or protect in the other than in oneself; an inner conflict is changed into an interpersonal one. Motivations, the wish for familiarity (König 1982), and easing of conflict, or the wish for communication with one who has similar experiences, can occur either separately or in various combinations. My desire for familiarity is satisfied if I experience a new acquaintance like an inner object of mine, or like myself. Thus satisfaction of a need for familiarity can come by transference of inner objects, or by externalizing parts of the self, as, for example, by the "narcissistic" choice of a partner. On the other hand, threatening object representations in conflict with the self are transferred onto outsiders for the sake of easing conflict. Objects threatened by inner conflicts can be "exported." In communicative projective identification there arises a greater likeness between the self of the patient and that of his target. A schizoid patient may thus assume that his target is like him, since that is his precondition for communicating.

In borderline patients, because of ego splits, various parallel ego states exist (Rohde-Dachser 1982). Such patients can shift their experience from one ego state to another, thereby eliminating conflict within the state just left. Projective identification can arise from any ego state: if it comes from one presently experienced, it can enhance communication; if it comes from a state not experienced at the moment, it eases conflict and promotes the split. It can support repression, too, in that the repressed material is experienced as lying outside.

Transferential projective identification (or transference with an interactional part) is the most mature form. It helps to establish familiarity but not identity, as in communicative projective identification. The other is assimilated to a familiar object.

If something projectively identified in the other is controlled, this does not necessarily amount to a special kind of projective identification. One does not always projectively identify in order to control another person, even if he experiences the controller's behavior as if the control were deliberate. What is to be controlled, that is, dominated, influenced, and limited, is what has been externalized from the self. That some other becomes the bearer of this externalization is inevitable but secondary.

Formations of psychosocial compromise vary in degree of definition. Among the more primitive ones are the basic assumptions of Bion (1961): dependence, fight, flight, and pairing. A more mature form of psychosocial compromise formation is the seeking of a scapegoat, which represents impulses and behavior defended against; an even more mature form is turn-taking. According to Bion, attitudes to basic assumptions and the fact of a group being a so-called working group are complementary. We disagree (König 1985).

The example of the scapegoat shows clearly how conflict easing as well as transferential projective identification can take part in an interpersonal process of intrapsychic origin. When one patient becomes a scapegoat by the others fighting in him rejected unconscious parts of themselves, one must ask why this patient and not another was chosen as the scapegoat. He may from the start exhibit behavior that corresponds to what the others reject. This may be impulsive, for example, arbitrary aggressiveness. On the other hand, the group may attack in this patient a defensive posture that they themselves show in a different, related form.

Perhaps, too, the patient may have been the scapegoat in his own family and thus shows provocative conduct that may make him the scapegoat in the group; more strongly than he would, were he not unconsciously seeking that role again. He thus transfers onto the group the members of his family that excluded, persecuted, or marginalized him, reverting to his role as a child. Formations of psychosocial compromise can be destabilized and changed not only by interpreting resistance and discussing instinctual impulses. They may change by themselves if the needs of individual members are inadequately protected by the compromise: those for whom it leaves too much or too little elbowroom will abandon it. Stock-Whitaker and Lieberman (1965) have described similar situations, speaking of enabling and restricting solutions of a group problem. Correspondingly, groups have norms with enabling or restricting functions.

Therapists and members can address interactional behavior. For example, one can show how a person causes himself to land in the scapegoat role, perhaps by breaking an implicit group rule. Tackling the interactional part of the various forms of projective identification probably acts therapeutically in groups where no or little interpreting occurs, such as self-help groups. Objects can then no longer simply behave in ways that meet the expectations of the projective identifier, because the interactional part becomes less effective. In the transferential case the transference is corrected because the objects behave not as expected. If, in the case of easing conflict, members do not behave as would befit the externalized parts of the self or objects, the conflict that has been made interpersonal must become internal again. Feelings of anxiety, guilt, or shame will return, and one looks for new solutions. In the communicative case the identifier finds that understanding becomes harder; he may feel misunderstood and excluded from the group. The consequent pressure of suffering can be therapeutically favorable if the query ensues, whether sameness of experience and feeling is really necessary for communication.

Chapter 7

Transference Triggers and the Course of Groups

Groups may be viewed as a complex system of transference triggers. The system consists of members, therapist, and the room in which sessions are held. Nonmaterial factors of the setting, such as time limits, have an influence, too. The system of triggers can be subject to many changes and can be perceived in different ways. Real changes, information about the group and the ego states of a member, as well as the kind of transference needs that in turn are linked with the state of the self, all bear on the effect of transference triggers. The sum of information about other members including the therapist grows in the course of the group process. In regression one often ignores information already at hand by denying or repressing it. Change in triggers by extra information does not alone set the group's run. We have observed that very short groups (say, five to eight sessions in a workshop for professionals) follow the same course as longer ones. Time expectations seem to influence perceptions in a group (see König and Sachsse 1981). The same kind of phenomena are found not only in group therapy but also in diagnostic interviews. Probably a small time concession will cause resistances to be retracted, which in turn may enhance exchange of information.

The peculiarities of transference triggers in a group make for faster and deeper (not necessarily stronger) regression than in individual therapy. Large groups regress faster and more deeply. Transference may fix not only on persons but also on inanimate objects, if they can be taken as symbols for persons, as, for example, the buildings and grounds of a hospital. A transference trigger is any perceivable item that sets off transference.

This definition is wider than that of Greenson (1967), who views transference triggers as an analyst's idiosyncrasies that distinguish him from other people. Several authors say that the group, namely, the members collectively, can be experienced like (not as) a mother in the various stages of a child's development (W. Schindler 1966), the pre-oedipal mother (Durkin 1965) or the mother as protectrix (Pines 1972), or as basic object for leaning on (Kutter 1971), but also the paralyzing, enclosing mother (Battegay 1975). If we ask what transference triggers can make the whole group appear in a member's unconscious fantasy as a mother, we discover simple facts. Compared with the group, the individual is small, taking up less space than the set of other members. The group indeed exceeds the size of each member several times, just as the mother is several times larger than the child. The group is several times stronger than each member, if we add their physical strengths (which are not used in a group but are potentially there), just as the mother is vis-à-vis a small child, particularly a baby. Moreover, everyone is both a member of and confronted by the group. This reminds us of the early symbiosis of mother and child, a kind of relation as described by Margaret Mahler (1968). If we say that this situation reminds us of the early mother–child relation according to Mahler, this holds in two ways: if you know Mahler's views, you will be reminded of them; but the situation can also trigger an experience similar to that symbiosis. It is the latter we have in mind when we speak of transference triggers here. In this symbiosis there are indeed already distinct interactions, as observations on babies have shown (Lichtenberg 1983, Stern, 1985).

The therapist, of either gender, is responsible for limits, among other things. If he sits down, a session begins; when he closes it, it ends. He gives the group and the mother–child fantasy within it a protected space. His task is to screen this space against disturbing external influences. In this function he resembles the father, at least the traditional father of our society, such as most of our patients have met him. Changes in the role of actual fathers produce variations today.

Freud (1927) stresses the protective function of a child's mother. In Freud's view only later in the child's experience does the father appear as protector. In fact, however, the father's protective role starts earlier in a traditional pair relation as most of our patients will have experienced with their parents, in that during the child's first few months and often long after, he shields the mother from demands and disturbances that might come from the outside world. Likewise the group in the therapist's room may feel safe under his protection.

We can pursue this analogy further: if patients' treatment is paid or subsidized by a health fund, the group therapist mediates between members and funds by writing out applications and reports. The fact that members' contributions help to finance the funds rarely plays a role in the patients' experience. The therapist works for the group as it were, by earning money for its existence, even if the fees end up in his pocket. With some of it he pays for the room, heating and cleaning and the like, which thus directly benefits the group. In speaking of the relation between individual and group, and individual (and group) and therapist, we here start from the simplifying assumption that the group as yet lacks a common history, so that members have no experience in common and little information about one another. We will show elsewhere (see p. 60 and p. 123) that there is a difference between patients and therapist to whom individuals turn and give information at the start. We will discuss changes through a history shared by group and therapist later in the text.

In early phases of the group, the maternal aspects of the group induce regression to an early childhood level of the mother–child relation and therefore a return to childhood. The therapist in his limiting paternal role at the same time enhances and limits the experiencing of that period.

In the early stages of group development, a member may feel small and dependent vis-à-vis the collective of other members, the "mother." He feels uneasy and anxious when experiencing conscious desires to break out of the group or the symbiosis with it, by taking on a leading position, while in later stages the fear of doing so may be linked with feared schizoid or anal-sadistic aggression or with oedipal fantasies of rivalry.

Regression grows with the number of members and their joint power, in two ways. If the member feels at one with the group (Scheidlinger 1964), he will see himself as protected by and strong with the others; if he finds differences and tensions between himself and them, he may feel weak and at their mercy. Such feelings when doubting the symbiosis are easier to take if a therapist is present to tell the patient what he as yet ignores, namely, that an adult can enter the childhood state but can return from it, too. Here the therapist's limiting power is greater than in individual therapy, for when a group session ends, not only do therapist and patient separate as in dyadic relations, but the group dissolves into its constituent individuals. With the mother group dissolving, the "mother" in fact ceases as inducer of regression. She survives only in the memory and the anticipatory fantasies of the individual, if he has developed to object constancy. Through such memories and fantasies the group's identity is preserved in the individual member while his regression diminishes when the group as such is not assembled. In the group we can reach deeper regressive stages and offer occasion for effective therapeutic work on early childhood relations, but we can just as quickly leave them again. Thus the patient may experience symbiosis but learn to emerge from it by a liberating process of development, learning to be alone in the mother's presence (Winnicott 1958) and in the ideal case to come out of therapy as an individual able freely to choose between associating with others or being on his own.

In deep regression, a patient is alone with the "mother" under the father's protection, that is, with a group of persons that merge into the single entity of the group. At other levels individuals remain in various social relations. With growing regression, these "more mature" levels recede from the perception of the individual, who then perceives the features common to the collective more clearly than what makes members different. In this stage of group development transferences onto the therapist have a relieving function for each individual: the therapist is a "lightning-conductor" for the ambivalent, libidinous, and aggressive feelings of the mother group toward the individual. We know the problems that can be caused in the development of a fatherless person when the mother aims too much of her libido and aggression exclusively at the child. In such stages of group development the therapist may be experienced as part of the mother group. Every growth in information changes the individual's perception, so that he will more readily perceive the other individuals rather than the figure of the group. This in turn acts against regression. Conversely, lack of information is a condition for regression caused by transference, which in turn limits the perception of distinctions and so diminishes the growth of genuine information, in a cycle of positive feedback. Lack of information in interpersonal relations furthers regression. Particularly in large groups we observe that the better the members know each other from earlier sessions, the smaller are anxiety and regression. Here anxiety is a consequence of regression: it is unnatural for an adult to be helpless and feel in a childlike manner. It is frightening not to know how strangers will react, not to be able to predict accurately or see how things stand, just as a small child often cannot reliably foresee how mother will react.

Along with growth in information, group development leads to a detachment from symbiosis, an initial experience of oral dependence, often aimed at the therapist. Later, when he has disappointed desires of dependence and members have recognized them, we reach an opposite stance that corresponds to the anal phase of the developing child: the group aims at autonomy and finally it becomes clear that the group contains men and women. Kinds of relation arise that include or are determined by difference in gender. The group enters the oedipal phase of its development. Who or what is the therapist in these various phases? He can be a father, as we saw; for example, even when he represents the reality principle and the group does not regress so far as to abandon recognizing that principle. However, he can be the mother, in cases where the feeling of helpless weakness caused by regression has become rather strong in the group and members experience the therapist as being stronger than all others together, partly by his remaining adult and not partaking in regression like the others. He remains adult because he goes on observing, distinguishing, and connecting, doing whatever belongs to diagnostic work, which helps to strengthen the secondary process type of thinking in the group by his secondary process type of verbalizing and conceptualizing. In sum he never gives these up in the same measure as the members do.

The therapist has more information about the individual members from prior talks and by having learned to draw inferences from observation and verbal behavior. That is why a session affords him greater gains in information than to the other members. If he is experienced as a mother, this is divorced from gender, just as a child can experience a male figure as a "maternal" caregiver. To the child at that age it means only that a person fulfills certain functions which in principle a man, too, can do—though, according to Winnicott (1956), a man may lack maternal empathy—so that he can replace the mother. This is true also of the developmental phase, in which the child experiences and recognizes the caregiver as an individual. A man, too, can be a caregiver and convey skin contact, interact playfully with the child, and give it the bottle. In the anal phase the mother is as authoritative as the father. In the phallic and oedipal phase the child learns that being man or woman is an immutable aspect of bodily shape.

At that stage it becomes important whether the parent of the same or the opposite gender had more authority in the family, because it affects identification with the gender role. Only at the matching stage of the group's development it becomes really important whether the leader is a man or a woman: if a man, a female member often takes on the role of mother; if a woman, a male often falls into the role of father. Only one member, not several, has this role, unless several compete for it, as happens in families where there is an effective constellation of mother/mother-in-law/grandmother or father/father-in-law/grandfather. In any case, individuals stand out in a specific gender role. Information about individuals is such that the group can no longer coalesce into a global object and defined social role relations become manifest.

All this holds for closed groups. In open groups things are less perspicuous. If a new member joins, this may trigger a regressive pull in a group that had previously reached an oedipal level, just as children can react by regression when a new sibling supervenes. This may indeed be therapeutically useful, since it enables members to experience this event in the group, while allowing the newcomer to witness regression that he would not have experienced if the group had remained at the oedipal level.

In general, a newcomer soon adjusts to the level of the group by adapting his perceptive level to theirs. In long-term open groups many conflicts are dealt with on the basis of an oedipal pattern distinguishing man and woman; these conflicts, sometimes from earlier phases, may be caused by induction, which occurs when a member raises a topic directly linked with earlier phases of the child's development (such as dependence or counterdependence, symbiosis or severance). By way of spontaneous staging (see p. 84) early forms of relation can thus be reactivated when within the group's pattern of relations a new member revives symbiotic, dependent, or counterdependent relations to individuals or the group as a whole.

The perception of transference triggers in a group depends not only on the transferential needs of members but also on the interventions of the therapist. One who aims his interventions at the whole group will direct the attention of members toward the group. Individual members will seem unimportant in comparison. Such a therapist gives the group a dyadic structure. A group of this kind will remain in the preoedipal stage longer than one whose therapist does not always interpret dyadically. Triangular processes, a precondition for oedipal development, will perhaps not arise at all.

Conversely, a therapist can from the start take up anything involving relations between three persons. Members' attention will then be directed to such relations, which hinders regression to levels of dyadic relations. In his indications, such a therapist will hold that patients with conflicts or disturbed development in the dyadic domain should not be treated in groups, while a therapist who favors dyadic structure may not accept members with problems in oedipal relations. The way a group runs can resemble a person's psychosexual development only if the therapist allows a spontaneous development by always starting from the surface of what comes up in the group, taking up dyadic and triadic phenomena when they occur, instead of forcing the group into a one-sided procrustean pattern. Reductionist behavior by the therapist may have many causes: his understandable wish to simplify complex group events, his own biography and personality, and probably the professional environment, in which preoedipal or oedipal aspects of psychodynamics are preferentially taken up and discussed.

Chapter 8

Countertransference and Transferences of the Therapist

In group psychotherapy we define countertransference as the feelings, fantasies, and impulses to act that arise toward individual patients or subgroups and the group as a whole. These feelings arise in reaction to transferences of patients and the group as a whole onto patients as actual persons and in face of the therapist's task. His character codetermines these reactions: on it depends how he reacts to a patient's arbitrary, dominating, or seductive behavior, but also acknowledgment or admiration. His character further determines in which group position he feels most at ease: as expert (beta), as follower of an unofficial leader (gamma), as a scapegoat (omega), or as one who initiates new action in the group (alpha) (R. Schindler 1957/1958 and Heigl-Evers 1978). There are therapists that are habitually alpha, beta, gamma, or omega. On the basis of his character, the therapist reacts to what the group offers, or he actively and unwittingly strives toward certain positions. Besides his character, the family constellation that is formed in the therapist's inner world of objects plays its part in the position that a member will aim to occupy. The therapist's current object relations with their possible losses likewise play a role.

If by definition we include in countertransference all feelings, fantasies, and impulses to act vis-à-vis the group, this will involve the consequences of the therapist's transferences onto the group as a whole as well as onto individual members or subgroups. For diagnosis, however, we must distinguish between reactions to patients as real persons and reactions to their transferences on the one hand, and the therapist's transferences on the other.

A therapist in a therapeutic group can aim at certain positions. There are corresponding cases in individual therapy: the therapist experiences himself as object in the relational domain of the individual patient and can desire to join him or an object mentioned by him. Thus the therapist can initiate new action in the patient's relational domain by remaining the expert or offering to be the scapegoat on whom the patient's aggressions are focused or whom the patient's relatives will hold responsible for all the failures in the patient's life.

The therapist can transfer onto the group an early maternal or paternal object and then react like his patients, although the cognitive tasks linked with his role as therapist usually prevent his ego regression going so far. He can develop transferences to an institution to which his patient belongs (a firm, clinic, or school). Equally, he may develop transferences in the field of the patient's object relations, such as his original family. By what the patient tells, the objects come alive and offer transference triggers. Still, they are usually not as effective as persons actually present in a group.

The therapist's countertransferences in reaction to transferences of the group as a whole and his transferences to it often become very intense. His task is to admit both but also to limit them and use them in diagnosis. In the psychoanalytic-interactional method, the therapist will selectively verbalize countertransferences, but usually not in the analytic and analytically oriented form of the Göttingen model.

Just as toward an individual patient, the basic transference to the group as a whole is often easier to diagnose if one imagines the group before or after a session than if one is directly engaged in the therapeutic process. As one gains experience, one increasingly succeeds in proper observation and diagnostic use of transference and countertransference in a group.

The therapist's countertransferences and transferences to the group become greatest if the group regresses deeply, or if it is very uniformly structured. This has the advantage that countertransferential feelings are not easily overlooked, although their high intensity is then a problem.

The greater complexity of group events as compared with individual therapy is a cognitive burden, the intensity of countertransferential feelings an emotional one. Because of both, few therapists regularly lead more than five weekly sessions of group therapy. Hence group therapy can never be a therapist's main profession, unless we include supervisions and scientific work on group therapy.

Countertransference includes reacting to projective indentifications by which a patient shifts parts of himself that his conscious self is in conflict with, or that are to be protected from attacks by other parts of self or by inner objects, into the therapist.

For some patients, projectively externalizing parts of themselves is the only way to communicate (communicative projective identification, see p. 34). The other members can function as a corrective to therapist behavior influenced by countertransference or his own transference. They may, for example, draw his attention to behavior that he unwittingly exhibits because it is similar to his everyday ways.

If archaic objects are transferred onto him, the therapist clearly discerns the feelings that the interactional part of such a transference and its ascriptions provoke in him. He then must avoid following the impulses to act implied in the feelings, which is not always easy if the feelings are intense. In deep regression, archaic qualities of objects transferred to and actualized in the therapist combine with a uniform experience of the members.

Regressed groups react more uniformly than less regressed ones. For example, a therapist who in a students' advisory center led a group consisting of depressive students disturbed in their work had the fantasy that he was surrounded by eight crocodiles, lying round him in the mud and intent on devouring him. The uniformity of a group's feelings, fantasies, and interactional behavior that mount up or intensify each other is doubtless one reason for what Battegay (1979) calls the emotional amplifier effect of a group; another must be induced feelings, as observed in fully occupied movie theaters as against almost empty ones: in a full theater people often laugh more loudly and weep more readily than in a half-empty one.

According to Racker (1953), we can distinguish between concordant and complementary countertransference. In the former, parts of self of the patient are actualized in the analyst, who then reacts with corresponding feelings that are similar to experienced or averted feelings of the patient (to be distinguished from the consciously desired identification with the patient's actual experience by way of empathy). In the complementary case the therapist reacts as object, experiencing the feelings that would cause an action familiar to the patient from transferred objects.

The therapist may indeed react differently to the transferring patient, namely, in terms of his own character. Just as in individual therapy, the group leader then reacts not to the transferential interaction, but to the ascription contained in the transference. He reacts also to the patient's behavior toward the transferred object, which must be distinguished from the transferential interaction. Thus a patient may try to provoke the therapist into becoming the strict father, then either rebel against him, obey him, or try to outwit him. This reaction of the patient to the transferred object summons up counterreactions in the therapist (König 1991b). Clearly, any behavior of the patient may trigger transferences in the therapist if the latter has had childhood dealings with people who behaved like the patient; for example, a therapist may transfer a younger brother who behaved toward him as he would toward a father. The therapist's children are inner objects, too, and can be transferred, so that he may react to the patient as to his own children.

As to transferences by the therapist onto the group as global object, let us recall that he knows quite a lot about each patient even before the therapy begins. This saves him from perceiving the group too much as a global object; members will only gradually catch up with him here. Still, therapists strongly disposed to transfer early objects can, like patients, blot out the differences between members. A therapist who has been a member of a training group will be more aware of such modes of reaction in himself and handle them better than one who lacks the experience of being a member. That is one reason why self-awareness groups should be part of any group therapist's training. He will thus know what it is like to be open in the presence of others and tell of things that one is ashamed of, or that cause guilt feelings or anxiety. There is a difference between telling this to a therapist whose professional role is to deal with such revelations in a helpful way or to fellow patients who do not have this task. They must not behave like a therapist or view the therapist as a bad model for openness, but as a model for considered use of their experiences in the group. In psychoanalytic-interactional group therapy the therapist acts as a model of openness, too, but within limits.

Although patients are all different, with different tolerance limits and domains of experience, therapists who have learned from self-awareness groups are less prone to misdose interventions in a group by ignoring the difference between openness toward a therapist and toward fellow patients.

By guided use of the feelings a patient evokes in him, the therapist enables the patient who reinternalizes the behavior and presumed experience of the therapist to work further through conflicts among parts of self and between these and objects (Ogden 1979, 1982).

Chapter 9

Neutrality as a Dynamic Concept

Every therapist is influenced by what goes on in a group. Beginners take up a rigid stance, while experienced therapists allow themselves to drift some way into transferential interaction and projective identification, thus enabling the patients to develop their transferences, as Sandler (1976) described for individual therapy. This has nothing to do with consciously playing roles.

What the therapist observes of manifest behavior by patients in the group is put into a different context, namely, understanding unconsciously motivated phenomena. This diminishes his emotive reactions and makes them easier to handle.

There is a difference between a child kicking someone in the shin and an adult doing so. If the therapist sees the child in the adult, he is better able to cope with the "kick," even if it is just as intense. One is less annoyed by a child and feels less threatened by him.

In sum, the better a therapist knows himself and his patients, the more independent and neutral his dealing with his emotions produced in a group. This does not mean that one does not wish to work with and help one's patients as real fellow humans: that one is glad if a patient improves and sad if he suffers; one is annoyed if he falls back into an old mode of behavior, and proud if he is successful, maybe even offended if he is not. Nor does neutrality mean that one treats all patients in a group alike. Parents with a big family do not give each of seven or eight children the same gift, but consider the degree of development.

Neutrality as a dynamic concept implies that the therapist can step outside neutrality. Such excursions are rarer, however, if he works at observing and understanding than if he does not understand his patients, cannot range his own feelings and so fails to contain them. The often cited mirror metaphor of Freud (1912) has done harm partly because a mirror is something undynamic.

Chapter 10

Working Relations

THE CONCEPT AND ITS APPLICATIONS

With the concept of therapeutic ego-splitting (Sterba 1934) (better yet, the concept of there being, in a therapy, more experiencing and more reflective ego states; see König 1991b), we can define resistance. A resistance is directed against progress of the therapeutic process. At personal and interpersonal levels, it is directed against the therapist and the healthy part of the patient's ego that cooperates with the therapist. It is directed also against the healthy ego parts of fellow patients with whom every member combines in the common purpose of advancing the group process and thereby progressing in therapy.

The working relations (König 1974b, 1985) are part of the real relations. Real relations are those in which one perceives another as he is. In transference relations one sees the other as in an earlier reality of oneself transferred to the present. Since we are never without earlier

experiences, there are no relations free from transference. Any relation has a real and a transferential component. Greenson (1967) sets
working relations alongside real ones and counts among the former a
mild positive transference (Freud 1914) functioning as a basic relation.
We find it more appropriate to regard working relations as real and a
mild positive transference as making them possible and supporting
them. The two kinds of relation influence each other.

Therapeutic ego-splitting can occur in various degrees. It denotes
parallel existence of different ego states, which alternate in their
influence on experience and behavior, and most people must first
learn how to achieve this. Whether they succeed depends on motivation, the ability to relate, and the ego functions already in place. At
the start of a therapy, therapist and patient enter working agreements,
but these can encompass only some parts of the working behavior of a
group. A large part of group norms that further therapy are implicitly
conveyed by the therapist through his behavior in preliminary talks
and later in the group: he takes up one thing but not another, and
treats some actions as resistance but others not. Where in his view
reality has been recognized, he stops analyzing.

We proceed to give some examples of norms that further therapy,
formulated as requests to patients and conveyed in part explicitly, in
part implicitly:

- Look at relations that develop during group sessions.
- Ask yourself why in these relations you experience in the way you
  do, what feelings and impulses to act arise, and how you behave
  toward others.
- Speak about your experiences and observations more openly than
  normally.
- Try to understand how feelings, perceptions, imagination, impulses
  to act, and action influence each other and how they relate to
  reality.
- As regards modes of viewing and questioning, follow the therapist's
  model.
- As to openness of your behavior in the group, avoid the therapist's
  model (holds for analytic or analytically oriented groups).

- Pay special attention to how together with others you try to protect yourself in the group against feelings of anxiety, guilt, or shame.
- When you have recognized this, try other ways of dealing with such feelings.
- From what you observe, experience, and understand in the group, draw conclusions for your ways of seeing things and your behavior outside the group.

This list is not complete, but the norms mentioned are numerous and complex enough to show that they could never be laid down as a working convention. Except for the request to behave more openly than elsewhere and to notice the relations that develop during sessions, these norms are mostly conveyed implicitly by the therapist during preliminary talks and group sessions, by what he takes up and thereby confirms what he can leave without verbal or nonverbal comment, or by what he discusses as resistance.

The main difference between the working relation in individual analysis and those in analytic group psychotherapy is that in the latter there are relations not only between therapist and patient but also between members working together. For example, patients notice when their own behavior is out of sync with reality and mention this, or call the attention of others to such behavior and seek explanations for it.

Working on transferences diminishes their part in relations, and reality becomes recognized. At the end of a therapy the patient should see the group conductor as he actually behaves in his role. The therapist's real behavior, even in the working relation, is the basis on which transference relations can be worked on. The behavior of the therapist should be consistent but not uniform. In the first session of a new group he behaves one way, and later differently. That a person's range of behavior varies according to situations is our common experience. The therapist with his range will remain an inner object for the patient, remembered more or less clearly, partly conscious and in time certainly growing partly unconscious or remaining so. We do remain active in the patient, even if he seems to have forgotten us. This is also so with group members. However, their roles are differently defined. They need not tailor their behavior as much as the therapist to whether it helps the development of fellow members. They can behave less reflectively and, as it were, more selfishly. They will thus be more critical and suspicious of the behavior of other members who, unlike the therapist, need not simply further the development of group members. Thus they will grant less of their implicit trust to fellow members than to the therapist.

In group psychotherapy, therapist and members must enable earlier relations to be renewed and worked on, but also offer forms of relation for which no prototype exists in the patient's biography. Therapist and members must be an adequately good mother (Winnicott 1974) who may not have existed, a triadic father who was lacking, or siblings a patient never had.

Therapist and members are subject to abstinence, though in different ways. Here, this means that desires for relations are barred from being always satisfied in the way they arise. Desire and realization should at least retain a gap, to further development. Besides, many such desires are tied to anxieties: it is precisely the prospect that a wish cannot be directly fulfilled that often prevents it from becoming conscious at all.

The therapist's abstinence particularly concerns incestuous desires. For an adult, physical contact can always have genital sexual overtones. Contact with a therapist who is seen as a parent could thus be fantasized as breaking the taboo on incest and have traumatic effects. Thus the therapeutically productive norm against bodily contact is vital in analytic therapy. In therapies that do not greatly foster transference, this may matter less. By contrast, many preoedipal desires for relation in the group are satisfied by the therapist and by other members at least in symbolic form, while the incest taboo should not be broken even symbolically.

As to assessing abstinence conventions, we note that in our culture bodily aggression among adults is inadmissible and must be transformed into verbal aggression. The latter is allowed to patients in a therapeutic setting. Sexual needs, however, are mainly met in bodily terms in our culture, even if they can be satisfied in more sublimated forms. This difference between sexuality and aggression in a therapeutic setting has not so far been much discussed explicitly. The therapist will have to observe when verbal aggression serves only to discharge drives and the aggressive patient does not intend to question his aggressive feelings and actions for self-awareness. In psychoanalytic-interactional groups the therapist likewise abstains: he talks about his feelings but allows them to determine his actions only as far as this seems to him of therapeutic use. He mentions only feelings of which he expects a positive therapeutic effect.

While the working relation with the therapist begins in the prior discussions, working relations among fellow members develop only during sessions. Still, even during prior discussion, the therapist can help to induce the patient seeking therapy to develop a wish to work not only with the therapist but with other patients in the group. Thus the therapist might point out that in a group what matters is to clarify relations to therapist and other members alike. In analytic group sessions the therapist is the example for the analyzing part of members' behavior; in psychoanalytic-interactional ones he is an example for handling his own feelings as well. In an analytic group he does not usually say what he feels and imagines, and he tries to limit expressions of his own feelings if he thinks that it might harm the therapy to exhibit them in the form that for him is ordinary; for this might have traumatic effects, or the scope of transference onto him might become too narrow through such information. In psychoanalytic-interactional groups he makes genuine if selective mention of his experience in relations with his patients.

To resolve misconceived transferences between members in analytic and analytically oriented groups, one uses more than interpretation. Since the patient is subject to less restrictive abstinence rules, he provides more real informations about himself; this helps to correct transference expectations. So, too, for a therapist in an interactional group when he names his real feelings.

Feedback via a patient need not as such amount to reality, a point that must be emphasized. Feedback may be distorted by transference; the therapist must make this explicit. This may not be easy, especially when a distortion is a precondition for satisfying the patient's drives (e.g., if a masochistically inclined patient perceives another patient's behavior as sadistic, because this allows him to derive a masochistic gain in pleasure, or if such a patient approves of real sadistic behavior and so enhances it). The feedback often becomes more precise if it comes from several members (performance gain of the group; see Hofstätter 1971). However, if feedback agrees between several members, the therapist may have to intervene if a subgroup or the whole group directs distorting transferences onto a single member.

Working relations must be strong enough for interpretation to be accepted. If such relations with the therapist are overrun by transference, he will have to deal with the latter first, before he can count on interventions being accepted. If transference relations are too intense, they can become intractable. If working relations occupy too much space, there will not be enough material that can be handled at that level.

The concept of working relations can be unconsciously misused by the therapist trying to use them in the service of countertransference resistance. He may thus prevent patients' transferences from becoming manifest, for example, by clarifying and explaining where it is not called for, seemingly to strengthen working relations but in fact to feed a patient symbolically and so avert aggressive eruptions. Considering the way norms for enhancing therapy are conveyed, we should see that the therapist, by the way he intervenes, cannot avoid giving hints on what he regards as important in the group and how the work should proceed. The reflection of this behavior via the concept of working relations makes it easier for him to recognize when and how he does this.

The development of mutual working relations among members is impeded if at the start of an analytic group the therapist interprets only relations with himself instead of including members' mutual relations. Moreover, members at the beginning of a group experience him less anxiously than they do each other. They know him from preliminary talks and can expect a supportive attitude from him. Interpretation of transferences when a group starts is often rejected as not relating to what moves patients consciously, namely, other members rather than the therapist. After such interpretation, members may object: "We hardly know each other; first we must become acquainted before we can attend to you."

Therapists who favor a more dyadically oriented view, in which a therapist relates to a group as if it were one separate being (e.g., Argelander 1972), will mainly value the working relations between patients and therapist. Group concepts, in which multiple mutual transference between members is taken as important, will give more weight to mutual working relations as well. If the therapist in an analytic group confines his interventions to relations with himself, this can reinforce the tendency that members can identify only with him as regards working relations. If he gives more attention to mutual relations between members, identification with other patients in the working relations of the group will be enhanced. Patients will hardly behave in an analytic or analytically oriented group in the same way as the therapist, namely, abstaining from talking about their individual feelings and fantasies. In individual therapy, too, a patient would look at himself as a therapist presenting himself as a therapist would present a case, but he cannot really analyze the therapist, who does not offer himself for this. By contrast, a group patient can analyze other members, without behaving like a patient himself, while the others may go along with this.

The concept of working relations differs from Bion's notion of the working group and basic assumption group as different states of groups (Bion 1961, König 1985). These states differ in the degree of members' ego regressions. The concept of working relations denotes various levels of relations with either the state of the working group or that of the basic assumption group prevailing, though not always in the sense of one complementing the other. Working relations and transference relations do influence each other, but their force at any time depends not just on the stage of ego regression of the group. Thus an intense working relation may exist alongside an early infantile transference relation, which leads to a considerable ego regression. This could be called regression in the service of the ego (Kris 1936). A strong working relation may even be what leads members to tolerate regression at all. Patients oscillate between an ego state more determined by transference experience and another more by reflection. However, transferential and working relations may both be weak since each depends on the kind and intensity of members' mutual relations as well as with the therapist, and therefore on the history of these relations in the course of the group, from initial motives that individual members bring into it, and on items in its environment.

THE THERAPIST'S AND THE PATIENT'S PART
IN THE THERAPEUTIC WORK

Though the therapist is protected by his technical knowledge and skill and by his special role, and most of the time is ahead of other members in grasping what is going on, he should try to enlist members as fellow workers.

Confronting as well as clarifying comments will often come from members themselves. In an efficient group, members point to each other's behavior, which they note in them and in themselves in reaction to the behavior of others. They actively try to discover what such behavior means. Their competence does indeed diminish in the sequence from confronting via clarifying to interpreting intervention. They can usually point out each other's manifest behavior, especially if it is repeated; they can clarify behavior and in discussion make its conscious and preconscious aspects transparent. They are less able to interpret unconscious aspects of such behavior, for they take part in the shared unconscious group fantasies. Often they are more regressed than the therapist, who shields himself from regression by his role of observer and preserver of his professional tasks.

In his protected role the therapist can be less anxious than the others, for he has decided beforehand to check his impulses and is not totally bound to bring them into the group by talking about them. He clarifies group events by taking part in them and works through the mass of material he sees in the group, using reality-related terms, vivid and accessible to members.

The therapist more than other members functions according to the rules of secondary process. A member who adopts a full therapist's behavior is resisting and prevents himself from being treated. Conversely, the therapist would be reducing members to infants if he did not let them take on some of the work of intervention (the more the longer the group has existed) as far as they are able to without harming active openness and free participation. A therapist has a delicate task in finding a balance between these two extremes.

What traits of the therapist might lead him to leave too little for the group to do? If he is a narcissist, he may fear that patients who take on some of the therapeutic work will come to be too like himself, thus undermining his uniqueness. If he is schizoid, he may fear that the patients may invade him. If he is depressive, he will give them insufficient scope if he wants to remain the group's universal provider. If he is compulsive, he may fear the spread within the group of attitudes and modes of behavior (indeed, a concept of behavior) that no longer agree with his own concept, so that he will constantly try to show how things should really be done. If he is hysterical, he might become afraid that members wanted to annex his analytic power. If he is phobic, he can counterphobically override his fear that his interventions might be harmful or intervene too little.

A therapist should make confronting and clarifying interventions if members seem unlikely to do so in the current session. Anyone used to working with groups will have experienced how often such interventions, if premeditated for future use, come from the group itself at the next moment. Groups heterogeneous in the psychodynamics of their members have the advantage that members' blind spots overlap only in part. A member may at times see as much as an experienced and analyzed therapist. The therapist may thus see himself as an all-rounder in a factory, who can temporarily replace a specialist. The therapist steps in where he spots blockages in communication between members, who cannot resolve this in reasonable time. Or we might compare the therapist with the master in a workshop, always lending a hand to colleagues or apprentices engaged in various tasks, without wresting the work from them; what he keeps as his own task is the overall planning and supervision of the work, taking into account the whole. He is particularly competent for interpreting modes of behavior that affect the whole group, psycho-

social defensive moves in which all members take part, and unconscious fantasies that he can infer from members' behavior. In this he
may, however, allow them to help him.

In what way is it right for the therapist to be a pacesetter? In the
way he deals with his own experience at the level of working relations.
He leads in grasping and working through events in the group. In an
analytic group he does not lead as regards open comment, but as
regards humane behavior and accepting what is bad or shameful in
others. In psychoanalytic-interactional groups he leads in putting a
group norm in question and when he behaves more openly than the
patients.

Work in a group should not be exclusively unpleasant and
serious. It is desirable for patients to welcome action and enjoy the
work, for all its unpleasant, frightening, and risky aspects in the group.

The group therapist has much to observe and do, even if the
group helps him in this. Freud (1937a) wrote in aphoristic hyperbole
that being an analyst is perhaps the third among impossible profes-
sions; the other two are bringing up children and governing. Group
psychotherapy is more difficult than individual analysis. The field is
more complex and the work emotionally more demanding, for several
reasons. Still, the group therapist shares with other workers the aim to
approach an optimum, not wholly to realize it. Like individual
analysts, and perhaps more so, he must remain someone en route.

Chapter 11

Resistance

In the complex group situation, resistances are much more varied than in individual therapy. Silence does not always mean resistance in the latter either (see König 1991b). Group members who remain mute can communicate nonverbally and a joint unconscious fantasy may arise. In a group, each can rely on another to start. Not so in individual therapy, where only one patient attends and either talks or not, with none to start if he does not. A group may intellectualize in discussion, thus turning the session into a kind of seminar. In individual therapy, the therapist will not respond in kind to such a style. In a group one finds interlocutors who do this. The convention of taking turns can exist only in groups, whether as implicit or explicit norm. Each member may at some time be the patient treated by the rest.

This structure of communication can be seen as a psychosocial compromise that arises during a session without as yet being a norm. For example, patients may deal in terms of one of them with a problem concerning them all. Likewise, we have psychosocial compromise when patients are ready to perform therapy in the role of therapists and not of patient ("eight therapists in a group of nine members").

As in individual therapy, patients may cling to the here and now, or speak only about external experiences and avoid topics in the here and now that would seem to be obvious. In jokes and anecdotes members may express themselves to the point, although such devices can also function as resistances. One who implicitly takes a therapist's role can ask and interpret. At times patients try this in individual therapy with the therapist, but in groups it happens much more often. Here members offer themselves more readily than the therapist who need not do so if he finds it inappropriate. A group may aspire to uniformity ("We are all alike or at least similar") and avoid or blot out variant modes of experience and behavior, or do the opposite: if new members join the group, new impulses may arise but so may resistances to integrating the newcomers, who are left aside by the others. Moreover, there is such a thing as overintegration, fantasizing, and demanding that the new members be like the old ones, to preclude change.

As in individual therapy, acting out can occur in or with regard to the therapeutic setting—some or even all members are late; sessions are canceled; fees are not paid on time; members may wish to smoke, eat, or drink and offer each other the wherewithal.

Some modes of behavior seem to promote therapy but are actually resistive. For example, if a patient reports a dream he assumes to be intelligible only to the therapist, he may be exhibiting a resistance to the group situation. He is seeking direct communication with the therapist while excluding other group members.

Resistances in groups may express themselves as to psychosocial norms and psychosocial compromises, as well as on the individual plane. There are as many basic forms of transferential resistance as there are possibilities of transference: onto individuals, subgroups, the whole group, the therapist. All norms that develop in the group are unconsciously determined as well. They can be ego-syntonic or not. Their resistive feature can be unconscious, preconscious, or conscious. Every group phenomenon can be seen from the viewpoint of norms or psychosocial compromise, as mentioned earlier. Resistive phenomena can have various functions. In turn-taking, members may work on another's problem that they cannot yet recognize as belonging to themselves. Further, they may select a member with enough ego strength to tolerate the working out of the topic. It may happen that members will select one whose resistances they know to be particularly hard to influence. The conflictual theme will then be worked on, but with the aim of showing that success is impossible. If taking turns has been established, there may be initial pauses of silence. Nobody dares to speak, because it would be his turn throughout the session.

Some patients are used to the scapegoat role from their original families and will actively seek it without noticing; in that case, the actual theme of conflict is less important. They will offer themselves as scapegoats in any context that arises. Seeking this role can thus be viewed as the interactional part of transference (or transference type of projective indentification): the person concerned unconsciously forces the others into the role of family members who in the past have excluded or rejected him. Still, tending to seek this role may coincide with the others' tendency to choose for it someone who shows a certain inner dynamic as expressed in his behavior. We distinguish forms of resistance that are more or less differentiated, the latter often having regressive aspects. Among them are Bion's basic assumptions: dependence, fight or flight, and pairing. Here we are dealing with fears that appear in regression, where members in the dependence state seek protection and shelter, refusing to become independent; in the case of fight or flight, something actual and endangered is to be preserved; in pairing, the pair is to yield something new, perhaps a savior of the group. Argelander (1972) has stressed the defensive aspect of Bion's basic assumptions. He also describes group cultures that resemble character structures: hysterical, compulsive, and so on. We can assign defensive mechanisms and resistive phenomena to group cultures as to the corresponding character structures of individuals, for example, displacement and trivializing as resistance in a hysterical structure, isolation from feeling and minimizing along with a tendency to make immobile in a compulsive structure, and so on.

Stock-Whitaker and Lieberman (1965) describe group processes as enabling or restricting activity, with resistances in restrictive group solutions coming out more clearly, though they also exist in enabling solutions. Interaction without any resistance does not exist.

All forms of manifest resistance can be therapeutically worked on. In the psychoanalytic-interactional form of the Göttingen model we preferentially address resistances that manifest themselves in the group's norms, in the analytically oriented form the psychosocial compromise formations. In the analytic form of the Göttingen model we alternately work in both areas, but more often find regressive forms of resistance, since the therapist's behavior here promotes regression more than in the analytically oriented form. Resistances have an adaptive function, namely, as brakes to the therapeutic process. Brakes are just as vital here as in a car. The speed of the therapeutic process must not exceed members' tolerance limits. If the therapist thinks that members are braking too hard and so stay too far from the tolerance limit, thereby inexpediently retarding the therapeutic process, he will address the resistances with the aim of resolving or reducing them. Members often help him in this. It may happen, however, that all members try to throw out the resistances, in which case the therapist has to brake by pointing out that members do not protect themselves enough.

When members come close to their individual tolerance limit, feelings of fear, guilt, and shame increase, as conscious feelings and also as unconscious signals that set off defensive mechanisms. If you consent to therapy and want to get well, you will generally be prepared to put up with some measure of unpleasant feelings. How intensely so depends on how strong the motivation is for therapy, and specifically an experiential one that sets off conflicts, which can entail unpleasant feelings. Optimally, patients feel their way as close as possible to the tolerance limit. The therapist, from experience with other patients, is sometimes better able to judge how much a patient can bear. Besides, he knows what positive effects can ensue from bearing unpleasant feelings and may try to push the patient into tackling more than the latter had at first intended. The long-term improvements a patient then gains may motivate him to go closer to the tolerance limit. Some suspected consequences practically never supervene in a group, or in individual therapy. Although members are not bound by the same abstinence rule as the therapist, they will often be less rejecting, aggressive, or indifferent than a patient had feared. Inner experience, too, may turn out less grave. Fear of fear and of feelings of guilt or shame is then not fully justified, the ego is not swamped by impulses, and the patient does not lose control. Conversely, all this may occur if the patient overtaxes himself, failing to protect himself adequately in the group.

Before a therapist can address resistances he must recognize them, which engages not only observation but also evaluation of group transference feelings and countertransference fantasies. The hypotheses derived from all this are to be tested on the observed and experienced group events. It makes no sense to address a resistance before it has become defined enough for members to see it. Here the therapist often has an advantage over group members. Impatience and eagerness to interpret on the therapist's part can prevent a clear emergence of resistances: members can be shown resistances, be confronted with them, only after these acquire a clear form. Early interventions by the therapist may, however, make a resistance more precise, for example, if members try to justify behavior that has been addressed and thereby make it stand out. It would be well for the therapist to become clear about the functions of any resistance, or at least conjecture them, before addressing it. However, this is not always possible; sometimes one must first confront resistive behavior by describing it and then see how members deal with the confrontation. One might, too, ask the members what is the value of resistive behavior and then jointly clarify the function of resistance. However, all this should be tried only if it seems likely that members taking part in resistive behavior can partly or wholly do without the protective function of resistance. That one cannot guess or know unless one has some view as to that function. If not, intervention must be very careful and gradual. Many resistances must be addressed time and again, but not in mechanical or automatic fashion; for resistances can change in function and a resistance that can be given up in one group session may be indispensable in another, to avoid crossing the tolerance limit.

To preserve its cohesion, each group seeks forms of resistance that equally meet the various protective needs of patients. Almost always some members need less protection than others. The first will charge ahead while the others will brake. For this reason the therapist must keep in mind the protective needs of individuals. Likely needs must be considered even at the setting up of a group.

To what role in a group a patient aspires, and what role will be assigned to him, equally depends on his tolerance limit. As we said earlier, the role of being a protagonist as to a particular problem, if the problem is to be elucidated, will be assigned by other members if the tolerance limit of the receiver is held to be particularly high, but also if it is held to be particularly low and his resistance is correspondingly high; if it is the patients' unconscious intention to show that the problem cannot be solved.

Every defensive formation in a group is under tensions arising from the various kinds and strengths of members' protective needs. With these tensions a group may deal more or less creatively.

Lack of skill in estimating their tolerance limit happens above all in patients with limited powers of introspection. Some are bad at assessing the effect of their behavior in the group and are surprised by how others, who cannot endure it, will react. Others perceive that their own tolerance limit is reached or even crossed, but cannot make this clear. Here the therapist must exercise his protective function and say, for example, that if he were in the patients' shoes, he, too, might find things unbearable. Sometimes he must bring members to see that they have overlooked subtle signals of the tolerance limit being crossed. Members may do this also, as when they insist on achieving something with a given patient but are afraid of feeling powerless in case of failure. In self-awareness groups tolerance limits are crossed when the participating therapists insist on being stronger than patients usually are.

We must distinguish resistive behavior from negative therapeutic reaction. In the latter, the patient responds to new insights and experiences by a decline in health not simply explicable in terms of overdosing. The patient might indeed use the new material positively but fails to improve because he must not. For example, he might begrudge the therapist success in an effective intervention; he may be afraid of having to end the therapy if he improves, so losing therapist and members; he may be averse to letting others influence him, which therapeutic success would prove had happened. Finally, he may feel a need to suffer, a well-known type of negative therapeutic reaction.

Homogeneous resistive cultures can arise in groups, especially if the patients are rather similar in structure. This needs to be remembered when the group is being set up. Such behavior is hard to influence, since the therapist then stands alone against the group's resistance and has to do without help from members who would incline to other forms of resistance than the one that is beginning to establish itself in the group, so that they take no part in it. In structurally homogeneous groups psychosocial compromise formations develop that are stable and hard to influence, an argument against such groups. Still, resistances in such groups often stand out very clearly, thus making it easier to confront members with them. A resistance may show in members rigidly clinging to certain roles in the sociodynamic distribution of functions. Like sticking to certain types of roles, this corresponds to a rigidity in individual defensive structures. If one questions a role position, this influences the holder's individual defense, and also the assigner's.

In the distribution itself specific resistances already appear. Thus patients who aspire to a group position of experts (beta) often tend to hold back emotionally and remain uninvolved; they often have compulsive structures. Patients who are habitual followers (gamma) will take no risks, as is the case with phobic patients. Habitually aspiring to leadership (alpha) can mean that the person concerned feels safe and comfortable only in that position and that he wishes to avoid meeting his insecurities. Such behavior is often linked with a narcissistic trait, or with a hysterical one. A scapegoat position (omega) will be sought for the reasons mentioned earlier, but also if the group member hopes to make narcissistic gains in the sense of masochistic triumph. Habitual followers shy away from risk exposure and seek a habitual leader for the sake of stable leadership. If members fear that interactions in the group are determined too much by feelings, they often choose a habitual expert (beta), who will help to keep discussion at a rational level. A habitual scapegoat relieves the other members by standing for disclaimed portions of the self, but also for a shared defense against having to deal with the rejected material themselves. Habitual experts protect the others from experiencing disappointment and aggression against the therapist, who does not fulfill the function of umpire in the measure the group wishes, so as to satisfy members' needs for safety.

A set of roles diminishes anxiety in so far as each member takes on functions that he is best able to perform, given the scope and limitations of his personality structure. If roles are put in question by interpreting their resistive function, conflicts arise: members become unstable and unsure. It becomes harder for them to keep out of group events conflict-provoking facets of their personalities.

In a hospital defensive structures can be more readily questioned than in ambulant practice, not least because the ward's therapeutic personnel often notice and catch aggravation of symptoms between sessions. Besides, the patients need not be in jobs, where failure to perform can lead to serious consequences for them and possibly for others also.

Much of the above shows the importance of timing of interventions in dealing with resistances. As mentioned earlier, resistances must be addressed when they can be recognized not only by the therapist but by the members, too. At the same time we must notice whether a form of resistance that has arisen and somewhat taken root in the group is at an optimal level (König 1991b). A group choosing a certain resistance may in fact be working optimally. If the resistance is put in question, it may be replaced by another that is more difficult to handle. One had best leave a resistance alone as long as the group can work with it productively.

The same is true for individual therapy. However, in groups it is often harder to assess what will happen when one addresses a resistance. Conditions are more complex. In the psychoanalytically oriented form of the Göttingen model timing is particularly important. A beginner often tends to address a psychosocial compromise formation as soon as he spots it, although the group can work quite well with it and members gain new insights and experiences. In the psychoanalytic-interactional form of the Göttingen model we have to note with particular care what ego functions, defectively developed or inhibited by conflict, a form of resistance aims to render dispensable. Resistance is then treated by dealing with the individual's defects of ego function and restrictions of object relations. The therapist empathetically identifies with each member. For example, he may show understanding for a schizoid aggressive mode of making contact in the form of an orientational swipe, but make it clear that he recognizes other forms as well and regards them as basically possible.

Norms can have resistive functions, but may also be too progressive and overtax members, for example, if the dangers of excessive openness are not perceived or denied and trivialized (Heigl-Evers and Streeck 1985). The therapist may introduce "more progressive" norms, but also "more restrictive" ones. He justifies them as alpha of the group, by appointing himself leader of an action that establishes these norms. In analytic or analytically oriented groups the therapist leads only at the level of working relations for dealing with what is experienced in the group, by reflecting and understanding. What marks an experienced group therapist is, among other things, the way he handles resistance in the group. This sets him apart from psychotherapeutically gifted patients, who can be quick to interpret resistances, but do this in the group too early and too often. In that case, the therapist has to act as the advocate of the protective function of resistances.

Chapter 12

Interventions

THE CONTINUUM BETWEEN INTERPRETATION AND ANSWER

Every reaction to another in everyday dialogue presumes a relational interpretation implicit in the answer. If we tell someone that he looks tired, we imply that our relation to him allows the comment and that we value him enough to tell him because we worry about him, and that he knows this and does not feel attacked but notices our sympathy. We may indeed be mistaken, as with any interpretation. He may think that we wish to diminish him or incite him to some action, perhaps a sexual one; to tell him that he looks tired may in fact be linked with such an intention. In that case, our comment assumes that our relation is such that he will feel diminished or incited.

Conversely, psychoanalytic interpretations contain statements about the kind of relation we have to a patient. An interpretation, for example, may rest on our assuming that we are related to him as helpers and that he shares this view, accepting interpretation as being thus intended, even if it can upset, disturb, or offend him. Moreover, the diagnostic assessment from which an interpretation is derived often, though not always, goes back to affective reactions of the therapist, which he cognitively digests; this part of his diagnosis need not be transparent (often it is conveyed implicitly).

Still, therapists are only human, and their interpretations are not always motivated by the desire to clarify and so help. An interpretation may contain an aggressive reaction to a patient, or be motivated by the desire to impress a patient so that he admires the therapist, and much else. These motives will be hidden in the inter-pretation, but the patient may spot them nevertheless.

In sum, any statement in everyday life and any utterance toward a patient lies on a continuum between interpretation and personal answer. Both are involved, though in varied proportion. Pure inter-pretation without an implicit position toward the relation is just as inconceivable as an answer without implicit interpretation of the relation.

THE OBJECT, FORM, AND CONTENT
OF INTERVENTIONS

In an analytic group we aim at correcting transferences by testing reality. Inner conflicts, by transference, become interpersonal and are worked on at that level. On reinternalization this will produce changes in the patient's inner world. A correction of transferences occurs when patients obtain information about each other and when the therapist confronts, clarifies, and interprets events in the group. These interventions are aimed also at the interactional parts of projective identification.

Confrontation draws the attention to something that is directly observable, while clarification is concerned with unconscious or pre-conscious aspects of behavior by relating what seems disconnected, preparing the ground for interpretation that connects conscious with unconscious material.

There are two types of confrontation. The first makes a patient aware of something. To a silent group one might say, "You are silent," but one could establish a preliminary connection by saying, "You have been silent since Mr. X spoke about his wife." This invites members to establish a link between their silence and the report by Mr. X.

The second type of confrontation, the only one apparently so called by some (Kernberg et al. 1989), picks out a certain aspect of previously clarified connections and invites members to deal with it further, for example, by saying, "It turns out that both men and women have said nothing after Mr. X's story, but perhaps for different reasons." This invites members to consider further the gender differences in reactions to that story. Confrontation and clarifications may alternate several times, until an interpretation is prepared. The interpretation may occur after clarification and confrontation, but it may have become so obvious that there is no further need to utter it; or it comes from one of the members.

The therapist may decide to leave it at clarification if he thinks that it is too early for interpretation, which had better come at some later stage. If a group is occupied with a theme arising from members' interpersonal relations, it will usually recur. Still, an interpretation may be given even without prior confrontation or clarification if one expects it to be directly understood and accepted.

Therapeutic interventions should start at the surface in either case. Their effect is then not just superficial, because the interpretation of derived conflicts can bring deeper conflicts to the surface. In regression, too, deeper conflicts come out and can thus be tackled. The therapist must, for example, watch whether a resistance in the group shows up more in the form of psychosocial compromise formation or as an agreement on norms. He will address first what seems to him nearer the surface.

Interpretations can be given all at once or gradually. The less regressed a group, the more complex the phenomena and hence often the more extensive the interventions needed.

Naturally, individual experience is more specific the later it figures in one's biography. Strong regression tends to unify precisely because early experience is relatively uniform, since small children are as yet limited as to refined perception and experience.

Interventions can be descriptive or metaphorical. Often it is expedient to translate metaphorical into descriptive language to attain a formulation in everyday idiom. This will provoke resistances that can then be tackled. The translation can be supplied by the therapist or by members during or after a session.

Group therapists who apply the concepts of Melanie Klein often use a language of symbols that circumvents resistances and directly aims at the infantile unconscious in metaphorical form. Such therapists usually spend little time on clarification.

Metaphor creates a distance between signifier and signified. Nevertheless, a metaphor can forcefully express what is meant, for example, in swearwords; it may equally express the meaning more gently, for example, as a euphemism. Metaphor leaves more room for interpretation than direct designation or description. A metaphor is vaguer than a description of the same content, but often conveys emotional links more directly and has the merit of brevity. Metaphors give access to metaphorical communication. Thus the metaphor of "Abraham's bosom" can be built up into a fantasy in which members are jointly in that position (Heigl-Evers and Heigl 1977). However, we may work cognitively, for example, by wondering who is meant by Abraham (perhaps the therapist). We thus go over to a descriptive level. After that we can continue working on the metaphorical plane, though influenced by having decided who is meant by Abraham. Translation into descriptive terms makes it easier to fix what is to be conveyed in the descriptive part of everyday language and therefore in ordinary life. As in Kleinian language, a metaphorical intervention circumvents members' resistances. Metaphor is often milder than description, so that protective resistances need not be provoked. However, if one avoids them and leaves them unattended, they impede the application in ordinary life of what has been conveyed by metaphor (König 1991c).

Interpretation, confrontation, and clarification are not sharply separate. One always observes something in the context of a situation. Thus confrontation already involves interpretation. Likewise, we cannot always sharply delimit clarification from interpretation.

A group's therapeutic potential is best utilized if the therapist first addresses individuals and gradually attains a group interpretation. In this process he can engage the other members. If a group interpretation is expressed, individual members will know their own part in group events as a whole, or they may reach such understanding more easily than if the therapist had deferred intervention until it had become clear to himself. Ezriel (1960/1961) recommended starting with a group interpretation and then explaining the kind of participation in group events to each patient individually. This is somewhat schematic. It makes little use of members' cognitive scope, in contrast with Foulkes, who is for therapy by the group and gave members a more active role in the finding of interpretations while he himself remained more reserved. Addressing individuals in the group is not as yet individual therapy in the group, if the whole is kept in view. Members' varied participation in finding an interpretation reveals much about the therapist's understanding of his role. By dealing with mutual relations of individuals, a common feature gradually becomes visible. Conversely, one can first address what is common and then let the group find the connection with individuals. If the group objects or simply shelves the group interpretation, there is resistance, unless all members actually react alike, for example, if an event of equal impact to all encourages members to such uniformity, or if a group is far regressed. Closed groups go through a development that corresponds to the psychosexual development of a child and thus react uniformly at each stage as regards the theme, though not necessarily as regards the way of experiencing and digesting it. Examples of events affecting all members are a member is late or stays away, the group has a summer break, there was some other break, a new member comes in or an old one leaves.

Many therapists shun addressing individuals in the group, since they think that this amounts to individual therapy in the group, which is regarded as a beginner's mistake. Leaving aside that one may wish to address one person and mean several, it is always better to pursue individual therapy in the group than to defer intervening until the session is over.

If the therapist spends much time with individuals, he emphasizes the differences between members. It counteracts the group's fusing into a global object and limits regression (see p. 91). One remains in the area of derived conflicts (Gill 1954). Whether it is therapeutically preferable to concentrate on derived or on basic conflicts depends on circumstances. If one lets the group regress strongly, it can happen that important defensive structures will be passed by. This will alter the basic conflicts but not the way they are digested individually. Conversely, sticking to derived conflicts may result in therapy touching basic conflicts little or not at all. At the surface something has changed, but at the core the old basic conflicts remain. Patients of hysterical structure are particularly prone to this. It may then be advisable to work in regression to reach the basic conflicts, when the hysterical mask is often shed.

If a patient is already overtaxed by his conscious conflicts, one obviously should not reveal unconscious ones as well. For individual therapy, Kernberg (1975) has pointed out that interpretation for borderline patients usually strengthens the ego, while for psychotics the opposite may occur.

THE USE OF RECONSTRUCTIONS

In individual analysis reconstructions ("constructions"; see Freud 1937b) serve to show a patient the genetic derivation of his present behavior. Once he sees how his behavior arose, he is better able to change it, in a transference relation but also in relation to persons outside the analytic situation.

One might ask whether in group psychotherapy it is reasonable to apply reconstructions. Many group therapists (for example, Ezriel [1960/1961]) confine their interpretations to illuminating transference here and now and report that just by doing this one can change a patient's behavioral structure. For individual analysis Strachey (1934) had earlier asserted that such interpretations are the most effective.

In catamnestic tests on patients who had undergone brief analytic therapy, Malan (1976) observed that the most effective interpretations were those in which one could also link transference behavior with persons who mattered in early development.

In group psychotherapy we use reconstructions if spontaneous genetic remembering is not to be expected, especially in the case of unconscious fantasies that can be derived from the developmental stage of the first two or three years. Moreover, we make sure that the reconstruction appears relatively "safe" in terms of the situation or the material previously brought into the group. Even then we do not state the reconstruction as necessarily true, but make doubly sure that the patient has scope to accept or reject it, for example, by saying "perhaps."

Using reconstructions in analytic group psychotherapy involves the technical difficulty that the therapist is dealing with several people: on the one hand, they all share a common unconscious fantasy; on the other, they do so in different ways, depending on their various biographies and structures. If the therapist offers a reconstruction, he has to keep it very general if it is to fit and address all members. If he tries to take into account members' different structures, he must address each member individually.

If he keeps to general remarks, this can tend to make members in the group feel neglected as individuals and sometimes produces anxiety. If he addresses individual members separately, he runs the danger of neglecting the collective aspect. For interpreting transference Ezriel solves the problem by connecting the relations the members desire with each other, and with the therapist, with relations that are avoided because they are supposedly dangerous ("calamity provoking"). By uttering the causal link between avoided relations and calamity, he distances himself from the necessity of this link and so enables patients to work through the fantasy of the feared link and to consider it with members in later stages of group development. As mentioned elsewhere (König 1973), Ezriel's interpretations are lengthy and thus interrupt the flow of group conversation, which in our view makes them less than suitable for constant use in group psychotherapy.

If one uses reconstructions, it is important to take individual members into account without neglecting what is common to them. We have therefore decided to adopt a technical procedure that is analogous to Ezriel's when interpreting transference in the here and now. Once we discern an unconscious fantasy in which all members seem to take part, we look for a common genesis of the fear that prevents it from being admitted into members' consciousness and stress this in our reconstruction, indicating briefly how this genesis may differ in individual patients.

A case by way of example: In an outpatient group the therapist had had separate conversations with all members, to discuss further participation of patients in the group and to gather further details toward applying for continued third-party payment. His announcement of individual talks had set off anxiety in all members about whether they would be able to stay on. The unconscious primary expectation process that group therapy would be available forever was undermined by the balance sheet flavor of individual talks.

At the start of the first session after these individual talks, which with one exception had shown that it was possible and desirable for members to remain, a woman patient (A) reported on insights she had gained in her individual talk and got the group to work with her on the problems that she now recognized. This showed her to be a "good" patient, who had drawn some benefit from the personal talk as well, but produced anxiety in the other members, who had profited less from their personal talks. The group discussion fixed on her tendency to be helpful to her friend, which revealed that she was afraid of losing him if she did not fulfill every one of his wishes. A male patient (B) then reported that he had lately realized he was not yet as advanced as he had thought, so that he was now resolved to consider areas of conflict of which he so far had no clear overview, especially regarding disturbances in his work, which were still present. He, too, showed himself as a good patient, working as a pupil along his analyst's line without as yet being able to reach him (the patient, too, would like to be a professional psychoanalyst). In this way he was trying to distance himself from his "therapist's behavior" in the group (repeatedly addressed by the other members) and subordinate himself to the group leader. Another woman patient (C) now mentioned that she intended to have an operation but was afraid that she might die under anesthesia. She was at the same time in the final stages of an individual therapy with a woman therapist and had there realized that she had a wish to die in anesthesia in order to have a swipe at the doctors. As several other members said, she was thus trying to exercise, or threaten, power through self-injury not only vis-à-vis the doctors but also toward the group and the therapist. At the same time she hinted that she had one other way out, namely, her individual therapist, whom she was going to visit after that therapy should she need a session; she was sure the therapist would not refuse her. When this theme had been talked about for a while, another patient (D) told of his work disturbances, which he could not put into perspective. He gave an intricate and apposite analysis of his problem, so that other members said to him that he really left no question open, but created the impression that he had grasped his problems; if anything remained unclear, he had not talked about it. After that the patient reported a variant of his work disturbances that consisted of his inability to accept other people's thoughts and concepts for fear that he might have to take them over completely and so lose his independence of thought. This showed that he wanted to be admired for his achievements by group and therapist, but that he was afraid they might make their own comments on this and raze his thought structures in favor of something else. The other members had taken part in the discussion in a way that suggested the problem had touched them personally, though it did not at once become clear how.

The therapist now gave the following interpretation: None of those who by their contributions determined the theme of the session feels that he can be loved and valued for his own sake. Perhaps this hinges on experiences from childhood. Patient A feels that she can be loved only as a kind of servant, Patient C that she can be noticed only if she is unwell or even dead so that others feel guilty, and Patient D that he is acknowledged only if he performs something outstanding, while he is afraid that his achievement will be destroyed. (Patient B was not addressed, since the interpretation that concerned Patient D partly applied to him as well and the therapist did not wish to address B's tactic of subjugation, lest B feel excessively hurt.)

The therapist went on thus: "Perhaps to gain her family's affection, Mrs. A always had to do what was asked of her, perhaps Mrs. C was loved only when she was ill and Mr. D only when he had done something great (at this stage, the therapist did not discuss schizoid fears of losing autonomy). Of course, people who impose conditions and make demands exist everywhere, not only in families. Perhaps you feel that I am doing this, too, except that power relations are different here. A child cannot live without parents, but adults have less hold on adults."

The interpretation was followed by genetic ideas from members addressed, not from early childhood but from later periods.

In the sequel, patients were able to state more freely than before how much they depended on the therapy, while the various degrees and kinds of dependence became clearer, in terms of what was real and what transferential. Reconstruction combined with pointing out the current reality enabled the patients to acknowledge and work on their transferential attitude toward the therapist (at first toward "therapy") less apprehensively.

DEALING WITH SPONTANEOUS REPRESENTATIONS OF SCENES INDUCED BY A STORY

Argelander (1972) described how patients' stories about outsider events represent the group's transferential state, which incites a patient to relate a certain event. The story has the character of a brain wave. Foulkes (1977) saw in this unconscious interpretations of group events.

In our groups we have observed the converse as well: a patient opens the group session with a story, and a constellation arises in which the group reenacts the tale, as it were. While Argelander's cases concern brain waves caused by the transference situation, our observations must be seen as analogous to the mirror phenomenon described by Heigl-Evers and Hering (1970). This arises when a control group of therapists watches a therapy session of patients and afterwards discusses it. The phenomenon can be observed also when a therapist reports on a session from his notes or when a tape recording of a session is played in a control group. If a patient tells a story in his therapeutic group, similar things may happen.

Following are some examples of this phenomenon of resonance, induced by a patient's story, probably explicable as arising from identifications. We will then consider how such phenomena can be utilized in therapy.

A woman student reports on the latest state of her marriage problems. She had met another man who seemed to be more understanding than her husband, whom she blamed especially for constantly wanting to have sex with her even when she was not in the mood. He accuses her of using refusal of intercourse as a means of forcing him into a certain behavior and "educating" him. She had hoped to be able to live with the other, more understanding man, but he did not turn up for a three-sided discussion, because the whole thing was too much of a problem for him. Next, the two men had agreed to talk it over without her, and she was now wondering whether she should ask the other man for a meeting. In any case, she wished to separate from her husband, at least for a time.

The other group members supported her plan by describing the advantages of independence, but then turned more to conflict between marriage partners as such and tried to improve their grasp of it. In this two men were particularly active, a male student of about 20 and a male trade-school teacher of about 40. The student wished to urge her on with interpretations that she could not cope with, so that she replied, "I am not listening." The older patient she was more willing to accept, as tackling her problems sensibly and really wanting to help her without staking claims for himself. Finally, the two of them spoke almost to her alone, then dropped their efforts, the younger one because he felt rejected, the older because he felt no longer able to summon up the understanding she had accepted and praised. The two men then exchanged their experiences on how they had dealt with her and tried to clarify their mutual relation, especially as to rivalry accompanied by the wish for rapprochement. A lengthy dialogue developed between them and the others listened. As for the woman student, she was "outside" as far as the two men were concerned. Here the therapist intervened by connecting the session so far with her story. He interpreted the young man's behavior as analogous to that of the husband who wanted to get her to establish a genital relation, transforming a mother–son relation into a partnership but being rejected. The older man offered paternal understanding, but felt unable to stand the strain. Finally, the two men spoke to one another, as in the woman patient's story, and she was excluded. To her, this interpretation was direct evidence, since in the group there and then she experienced with others a behavior resembling that of her two partners, so that she had to conclude that since the same might happen to her with others, perhaps she had some part in the marital conflict that she had not clearly seen before. The two men, along with the other members, then worked on the way she saw partnership in the primary group of her family and in the current case.

The emergence of the phenomena described in a therapeutic group enables the leader to interpret scenes of special evidential force, since the link between group events and a patient's story can be made directly apparent. In this way one can clarify a set of relations in the group. Patients cannot easily avoid the evidential character of spontaneous representations induced by a story, and fruitful disturbances can arise. Still, we hold that such representation can be made permanently fruitful only if the problems so revealed are worked through in the sequel and so made retransferable to everyday life. In some cases it may be difficult to distinguish transference notions (induced by a transference situation of the group) from stories that set up a certain relational situation in the group.

A story at the start of a session can, of course, be induced by the transference situation in the group; conversely, there must be a certain readiness in the group to represent in a spontaneous scene a situation described in a story. What influences this disposition is the prior state of transference, the position of the storyteller in the group, and the way he or she tells the story. A member in a marginal position will find it harder to interest the group in his story than a central member; however, a member who has been silent for a long time can attract the group's attention precisely because he speaks rarely. This is different from a supervision group that meets with the explicit aim to deal with a specific problem, for instance, a demonstration session of a patient group, a therapist's report, or a tape. As a rule, one will be dealing with the phenomenon we mean, when a member tells a story of such importance to him that he offers it expecting help from the group (the story is then not just a notion within group events but clearly an account of a problem brought into the group from outside). Moreover, we have observed that this phenomenon generally occurs only when a member could tell his story in one piece and keep the group's attention; this, too, is similar to supervision, where a connected input is provided.

If a therapist one-sidedly favors the group events in the here and now, he will view and interpret a patient's long connected story about external events as a resistance. The members' attention is turned from the here and now to the outside and the past; a patient's story to which the whole group attends prevents interaction of members mutually and with the therapist. With this we should agree if a patient always talks only about the outside and not about his experience in the group. In trying to decide whether resistance shows by telling a story about outside conflicts or on the contrary by keeping silent about them, which, of course, may also be the case, empathic identification with the teller can be helpful, with special attention to the emotional content of the story.

The interpretation scenes set off by a story must be used sparingly and only in cases in which one can expect strong evidential experience for both teller and group, with scope for making the experience fruitful at the group's current stage of development. There is then no danger of excessive interpretation of induced spontaneous scenes, thus inviting stories about outside conflicts beyond what is of therapeutic use.

DEALING WITH DREAMS

How few or many dreams are told in the course of a group therapy strongly depends on the therapist's position on them. One who regards the telling of dreams in the group as merely a resistance will usually address it as resistive and thereby brake it. One who tends to turn a psychoanalytic group into a dream analysis with spectators will encourage the production of dreams to an inflationary degree.

That dreams in a group express resistance is argued for as follows. Dreams are intimate phenomena that belong to individual analysis (a therapeutic relation between two persons). To introduce them into a group means that the teller seeks a relation with the therapist that more or less excludes the others, since the therapist normally has the best grasp of dream language. Thus a person who tells a dream in a group may wish to avoid conflictual relations with the other members. Further, to tell dreams in a group is therapeutically impractical, because time is usually too short to work regularly on all members' dreams.

In favor of the view that dreams in a group can be useful for creating access to members' individual unconscious, the following arguments are urged: A group is a good resonator in which a dream can be made to "sound." In the refraction of individual members' notions and reactions, a dream gains special clarity in the tension between manifest and latent content, which gives expression to current group conflicts. Even if no group conflict shows up in the dream, it is therapeutically valuable to tell dreams in the group and to work on them. One member's dream can throw light on the group situation and so become effective for each individual, without each being given the opportunity regularly to tell his dreams.

As regards dreams, we adopt an intermediate position. During group therapy, as in individual therapy, members may remember dreams and wish to understand them. To always address the telling of dreams in a therapeutic group as resisting conflict inside the group would amount to treating it as acting out in the group, a form of resistance that should always be addressed first.

The way an individual deals with himself in a dream has its place in a group, along with talk about conflictual experiences and relations, whether outside or inside the individual. Dreams can be treated like fantasies that a member brings into the group. Dream analysis arose from one person, Freud, talking to himself as it were. By transposing this to a relation between two, the therapeutic use of dreams has developed from an analysis of inner conflicts of instinct and character to analysis of the transference–countertransference relation as well. Dealing with dreams has shown us that individual dreams can readily lead to deeper explanations of conflict in a group, though not always and in all contexts. This is the area of the phenomenon of so-called group dreams, which often reveal an inner discussion of a member with the group even at the manifest level, and thus throw light on relations in the group from a new and so far unadopted perspective.

Given these reflections, the therapist, in his preparatory talks, can state that a patient may report dreams when he thinks of them, when the question is what may be mentioned in a group. The way the therapist later deals with dreams in the group will make it clearer still what scope he will allow them.

As a rule, the therapist can tell from the way dreams are introduced whether the resistive aspect is prominent or not. As always, he will have to decide whether to address the resistance at once. We find that great importance attaches to the "introductory formula" of dreams and the manner in which they are raised by a patient at the start of a session or in the course of it.

A member started a session, after strong rivalry disputes in the previous one, as soon as the therapist entered the room and before he had really sat down. Under clear eye contact with him, he said: "I wanted to start this session and tell of a dream, before anyone else starts talking." There followed a dream of a hike with his father through meadows and fields.

The introductory sentence alone suggests to the therapist that the other members are being shut out. The content of the dream may be linked with a wish to merge peacefully with the mother group dreamed as a landscape, in the therapist's company; here members as individuals would be in the way.

Another example: In the fifth session of a psychoanalytic group meeting every two months on weekends, a woman member who had never yet spoken first began after a longish silence: "After four sessions last night and this morning I am tired and wanted to just listen, hoping that someone else would say something, but it now seems to me that I must start things rolling. Let me tell you of a dream I have had repeatedly for months. So far I cannot do anything with the dream. Perhaps you could give me your ideas." This introductory formula makes clear that one must watch the role this patient wants to assume in the session. She is saying that she feels responsible for the progress of the group and gives this as the reason for her activity.

Every dream told in the group must be related to the context if the manifest content and the group situation seem at first blush unconnected. An example: A woman states, "I am dreaming that my teeth are falling out." She tells the dream in the following group situation: members have for some sessions been talking about feelings of shame experienced when realizing the gap between their own ideal self-images and their real possibilities. To see oneself as mirrored in others provokes shame. The therapist now looked for a link between the dream and the group process.

Any dream can be understood both as individual and as relating to the members, who, for example, learn about teeth dropping out in the woman's dream. Dentists report on their patients' feeling of shame when losing teeth. Of course, at an oral or oedipal level the dream may refer to still other fears. It may also mean that other group members will turn away from her if they knew her "from within." The group members' answers to her tale and the way she deals with it must be noted and dealt with therapeutically before the dream's content.

A further example: A woman member tells a dream, and the members one after another tell theirs of the night before. To the therapist it seems that the members are "diving" to pass below their rivalry for him as yet manifest in the previous session. In the dreamers' contest this rivalry still remains recognizable.

Obeying the therapeutic rule "Resistance before content, analysis from the surface down" (in the conditions of applying psychoanalysis in the group) and observing the links between manifest dream content, latent dream idea and the mutual relations of members make possible a sensible use and working on dreams in an analytic or analytically oriented group therapy. For the rest one observes time and again that there is "no time" for dreams in a group if members' energy and attention are absorbed by frequent manifestly conflicted relations.

In analytically oriented, and even more in psychoanalytic-interactional, group therapy of the Göttingen model, one must note how dealing with dreams can foster regression and sometimes limit oneself to working with the manifest dream content if it looks as though a regression is in the offing that is therapeutically undesirable at the time. This may happen in analytic group therapy, too, but more rarely.

DEALING WITH REGRESSION IN ANALYTICALLY ORIENTED AND ANALYTIC GROUP PSYCHOTHERAPY

In analytically oriented therapy in the Göttingen model one works with derived conflicts (Gill 1954) and their attendant impulses and defense mechanisms. The phenomena involved are complex. The therapist does not greatly foster regression, so that he can remain at the level of derived conflict. In psychoanalytic group psychotherapy, in contrast, the therapist will promote regression more, so that the basic conflicts come to the surface. These phenomena, relatively simpler in structure, are more marked, so the field of observation is less complex.

The regressive level can be influenced by the frequency and content of interventions. If the therapist intervenes little and allows long silences, speaks in hints rather than descriptions, and remains fairly aloof, regression is fostered. If he intervenes more often and does not allow such long silences, speaks more explicitly, and behaves more openly, less regression will be induced. Conversely, the phenomena being more complex in a group that regresses little, interventions will be longer: this follows from the complexity of phenomena in psycho-analytically oriented group psychotherapy. Such long interventions are a brake on regression, in contrast to short and more allusive ones because they will reveal more about the therapist.

While in analytic group psychotherapy the stress is more on shared features and one speaks more about the group than about individual patients, in psychoanalytically oriented group psychotherapy one emphasizes differences in experience and behavior of members.

In psychoanalytically oriented group psychotherapy one can profitably use interventions directed upward, that is, ones that address adult aspects of experience. For example, the patients fantasize about lying on a lawn. One of them says that he once had spent three days at home mostly stretched on a couch, almost never getting up. The therapist says, "You would all like to go on a vacation." He refers to a situation in which regression can be tolerated quite well, because it is limited in time and no work needs to be done . A clear temporal limit of a session results in regression being experienced as less dangerous, because members know that the session will end at a set time. They can abandon themselves to regression without too much fear.

MODE OF WORKING OF THE THERAPIST IN PSYCHOANALYTIC INTERACTIONAL GROUP THERAPY

While one can regard analytically oriented group therapy as psychoanalytic, with the therapist trying to prevent the group going into deep regression so that more mature forms of psychosocial compromise (and not the basic assumptions of Bion [1961]) prevail, psychoanalytic-interactional group therapy differs more strongly from the analytic type. The therapist takes a different line with the same material that for patients with a more robust ego he would interpret. He does not interpret, but "answers." In this he is selective, unlike a patient in an analytic group who is to speak about his own feelings. However, in a limited way, the therapist is then a model not only for dealing with what is experienced and learned in the group but also for conveying feelings.

Part of therapeutic procedure here is to confront patients with disturbances in their ego function (Bellak et al. 1973), when they are shown how behavior thus disturbed strikes an interlocutor. At the same time this puts in question the kind of current object relation.

Certain kinds of object relation result in ego functions not being available because they have been immobilized by some relational fantasy. Conversely, certain archaic fantasies about object relations and corresponding experience and behavior can be fostered if certain ego functions (e.g., ample reality testing) were not developed. By making himself available with his real experience, the therapist makes possible a correction of transferences without interpretation. In the same way, fellow patients correct transferences in an analytic group by speaking about their actual experiences.

The therapist might state how he would experience and perhaps even act in the patient's place, or in another member's with whom the patient has links. He thus assumes an auxiliary ego function, exhibiting alternative possibilities of experiencing and acting, or confronting the patient with various possible outcomes of his actions, which complements his perception and judgment. This gives the patient a better view of how his behavior will strike others. In this one must avoid creating the impression that in a given situation there is only one "correct" way of reacting. The intervention must be formulated with care. If one says, "In your place I should feel and act thus and thus," a patient will assume that the therapist means the advice to be adopted or developed as "correct." If the therapist says, "In this situation I should feel or act thus," he leaves it open whether he himself would react in this way or whether he means that he might do so if he were someone like the patient.

The therapist should always be alive to the variety of character structures, which leads to a variety of experience and behavior, and that one cannot decide which characterologically determined experiencing or acting is "correct." Alongside this variety we have extreme forms of character structure that are the rule in severely disturbed patients and must be considered as pathological. Here the therapist should be clear whether he is to intervene as himself in the patient's shoes or as an empathizer. If the former, he runs the risk not only of representing his experience and conduct as the only correct one, but also, since he tends to be healthier than the patient, of showing the latter an unattainable ideal of normalcy and health that leads to resignation rather than further development. In patients with structural ego troubles, what is disturbed in various ways is the ability to introspect, to tolerate feelings and control impulses, to shield oneself against stimuli by adaptive and selective perception, to foresee the effect of one's own conduct on others, and to admit regression in the service of the ego (Heigl-Evers and Heigl 1983). The ability to introspect is restricted if there are strong tensions that one prefers not to confront, or if inner conflicts are warded off so that the inner world appears "uninteresting." The patient has a feeling of inner emptiness and no motive for dealing with it. Tolerance of affects and impulse control are disturbed if corresponding structures in the ego were not built up. This happens when during development there were no or few interactions able to foster it. Being unable to ward off stimuli is a general sign of an immature ego and hinges on how mature are our representations of self and objects. A defective ability to regress for the sake of the ego is linked with a defective tolerance of affect and impulse control. Affects may take hold of the ego in all domains leaving no room for reflection. A lack of impulse control results in fear of impulses to act linked with regression. The effect of one's own actions on another cannot be foreseen if there is no relevant experience of specific interactions or when a symbiotic fantasy rules relations. Dealing with the other will then be viewed like processes in oneself: "He knows what I think of him, how I experience him, and what I fear in him." If ego functions are underdeveloped or paralyzed by conflicts, interpersonal relations are impaired. Current experiences become internalized and modify inner objects, which can thus be pathologically stabilized and deformed into archaic caricatures.

Likewise, the interactional part of transferential projective identification helps to stabilize the inner object images, these being constantly confirmed by interpersonal experiences. Successful communicative projective identification promotes the illusion of broad communication between self and objects.

The interactional parts of the three types of projective identification can be confronted by the therapist or by the other members. The patient notices why he repeatedly has the same experience, which until now he had not so far ascribed to his own conduct, but to the others reacting in a certain way.

If a patient has learned to bridge his difficulties in object relations by some compensatory conduct, it should be suggested to him that he is perhaps compensating; here one will often have to cross the boundary to interpretation. However, it is often best at first to address the drawbacks of compensating behavior. A counterphobic patient who deliberately courts danger because the attendant fear is more bearable to him than the taunt that he is afraid (König 1986b) can be reminded of the dangerous nature of his conduct. In other cases, too, compensating modes of behavior are often important for self-esteem. They must be regarded as abilities of which the patient is proud. This makes it hard to work on them.

If the problem is to clarify connections between a defective ego function and the underlying object relation, one will have to interpret, either implicitly or explicitly. The narcissistic offense will diminish if the therapist says that in some situations even he compensates, for example, by growing at first more polite when he gets annoyed with someone.

As Heigl-Evers and Heigl (1983) have emphasized, it is vital for the therapist to be able to empathize with the patients' needs for specific object relations. This enables him to signal acceptance and so make confrontation more bearable, and creates a model for not having to find another person totally good in order to accept him: one can empathize relational needs and understand them while wishing that they would change.

Therapists might even introduce personal experiences about the slowness of change in behavior, as Heigl-Evers and Heigl (1983) suggest. This makes it easier for the patient to accept that progress is slow and setbacks can occur. Moreover, these authors suggest that mentioning learning progress in the sense of Heigl and Triebel (1977) or Blanck and Blanck (1974) may be useful.

An important way of intervening in psychoanalytic-interactional group therapy, equally applicable to the other forms of the Göttingen model, is clarification of affects. The therapist, suspecting that the patient has certain feelings, gives him their names, or speculates on what he himself might feel in the patient's situation. Here, too, it is vital to stress that one is not the same person as the patient. If the patient cannot experience the feeling concerned, he might react to such interventions like a mystified child, as when parents wanting the child to go to bed try to pretend that he is tired when he is not.

We mentioned before that a patient may experience his ego as "empty" because conflicts are being warded off. Affects caused by the conflicts become too strong for the ego to bear. If translated into action, the result might be catastrophic. As with reconstruction upward, the therapist can intervene by naming affects and impulses to action that will be socially adequate. This sometimes enables a patient to admit a more intense feeling of the same kind, as long as he is aware that there are "more adult" ways of reacting to those feelings than the ones he fears. If corresponding affects and impulses fail to become conscious, structures for dealing with them are nevertheless prepared. These will be tentatively available if, for example, in a later analytic therapy resistances are resolved by interpretation, thus releasing impulses that the patient is at first afraid of in everyday contact with others. Here, too, we must beware of presenting an unattainable ideal of normalcy, which tends to discourage the patient rather than helping his development.

In patients already overtaxed by conscious conflicts, resistances against unconscious conflicts becoming conscious should not be addressed at all or only with great caution. This holds for the patient's psychosocial compromise formations as much as for his individual defense mechanisms. More useful for therapy in such cases is to question normative regulation of conduct (Heigl-Evers and Schulte-Herbrüggen 1977, Heigl-Evers and Streeck 1985) a group "negotiates" (Streeck 1980). The norms of a group can leave more or less free room: reducing it has a protective function but brakes development. Functional defects in patients with disturbed ego structure enter the negotiated framework of norms. Such defects may cause patients to assume free room to exist when it does not. Heigl-Evers and Streeck (1985) give as an example a group in which the norm developed that members should show unreserved mutual trust, the result of a reciprocal primitive idealization of members. The therapist said, "I am not too sure; when I look around, and imagine I entrust myself without reserve, I do feel a bit uneasy, for I do not know what I would have to expect from every one of you." Here the therapist mentioned the norm and at the same time stated that he did not accept it. By expressing his uneasiness he wanted to make the norm relative and draw members' attention to how relations in the group were in fact constituted. Later it became clear that members who had remained silent during the discussion on norms would not have reacted favorably to absolute candor.

In another stage of the group's development, paranoid notions might have predominated, perhaps with the norm: one should not be open, because this always leads to trouble. Here, too, the therapist could convey from personal experience that openness does not always and everywhere lead to trouble. He thus would point out that there might be more free room than the norm suggests. When his task is to alter norms, the therapist initiates action. He then is in an alpha position, which he should not aspire to in the other two forms of the Göttingen model, except perhaps in working relations. The therapist may be attacked for his suggesting norms; if so, he reaches an omega position, as an inner opponent of the group, but can regain the alpha position of a leader. Like all psychoanalytic procedures, psycho-analytic-interactional therapy is being further developed. This involves important questions: How can a therapist, by offering relations, best promote the internalization of an object ensuring the building up of effective ego structures via identifications? Is it always necessary that the therapist name his feelings? When is it enough to express them nonverbally?

Many patients with disturbed ego structures are weak in decoding nonverbal feelings of others who convey them by mime or gesture. With such patients it may be useful for the therapist to name his feelings. Besides, a patient may find it hard to link such names with something concrete, especially if he cannot yet name these feelings in himself. The names then have no substrate accessible to him. With such a patient the therapist should perhaps first try to clarify what a patient feels and to make his feelings more vivid and manipulable by naming them as in clarifying affects. In the sequel the patient might then be able to make more of the therapist's feelings.

Doing research on members of psychoanalytic-interactional groups, Ott (1991) has shown that they found it less helpful if the therapist named his own feelings rather than trying to clarify those of members. These members, however, had no severe defects in ego structure, but perhaps the difficulty of naming one's own feelings is quite generally underrated. Difficulties of members in psychoanalytic training to name their own feelings in connection with the diagnosis of countertransference point in the same direction.

Maybe, too, we should be more aware that what determines a therapist's action are not only feelings like curiosity, anger, and sympathy, but also his therapeutic goal. In asking for information, he might be curious, but more likely he pursues his task, for example, by trying to grasp a patient better. Here it is neither necessary nor useful for the therapist to link a question with feelings of curiosity that he may indeed experience but which are not his main motive. Many patients will more readily accept that a therapist wants to know something from them if it is from a therapeutic attitude rather than from curiosity.

Chapter 13

Group Therapeutic Concepts and Handling Them in Practice

A therapist deceives himself if he thinks that he is only interpreting, or, as in the Göttingen model of psychoanalytic-interactional therapy, only "answering." This is confirmed by Davies-Osterkamp and colleagues (1987). It became clear that Heigl-Evers as a therapist in such groups interpreted more often than the concept stipulates, while in the psychoanalytically oriented form she answered more often than she herself seemed to notice. With therapists who, unlike Heigl-Evers, do not apply a concept developed by themselves, the gap between theory and practice is no doubt greater still.

One can regret such discrepancies, but one can use them positively, too: in practice the demands of therapeutic work assert themselves in that a therapist will take some needs of the patients into account and adapt his conduct to them, even if his concept does not provide for it.

The fact that experienced users will overstep the limits of some concepts and achieve favorable results (we have indeed found this with colleagues who thought they were making "scholastic" use of certain concepts) leads us to recommend this in practice. For teaching certain procedures it may be at first better to insist on respecting a concept, but only as a central guide on which therapeutic work should concentrate without being confined to it. However, the therapist must not attend to too many things at once, since he cannot keep in view limitless numbers of connected phenomena at the same time. He can, of course, see or perform different things in sequence, looking at various aspects of the therapeutic process one after another. He can work with the here and now, with outside relations, with occurrences in the patient's past, now interpreting, now answering, mainly address the group as a whole in relation to himself or members' mutual relations, or temporarily perform individual therapy in the group.

This does not mean that everything goes. A therapist should not behave in an arbitrary manner, but we do favor varied and flexible conduct. He should know why he acts as he does or at least be able to give plausible reasons for it afterwards. In a therapeutic situation one will sometimes sense the reason rather than mentally formulating it; the patients should perceive that the therapist behaves in a richly varied way, adjusting himself to the circumstances and competently dealing with them, not from boredom with always doing the same thing, at times found in capriciously hysterical therapists, who thus frighten and irritate patients.

Part II

Special Practices

Chapter 14

Behavior of Therapist and Patients Specific to Structure and Transference

In a group, a patient remains silent more often than in individual therapy. A member can always let the others talk. Some schizoid patients keep quiet for long periods. Though not yet ready to take part in the group's verbal interactions, they do take part in the group process by identifying with other members. Through information that they gain about other members they correct initial misperceptions due to transference. They can make much progress even if silent (König

1975c). Not so in individual therapy, where the patient has to speak without a therapeutic process in which to take part silently. In remaining silent, such patients can sort out what they wish to take up, by selectively focusing their perception. The other members tolerate their silence because they feel that the silent ones are taking part this way but are unable to do more. The therapist must ask himself whether the patient's silence is internally productive or shows a resistance to be dealt with. From the early days of our own work in group therapy we remember a patient with obstipation and abuse of laxatives who, after some sessions in silence, stopped her therapy. Here the therapist should have intervened. This case brings out a decision problem for the therapist: whether or not to address silence. There is adaptive silence and communicative silence in which non-verbal signals create a group fantasy.

Not all patients with early disturbance remain silent. Some, of borderline structure, try to produce group situations in which they rediscover split objects: there are individual members or subgroups they identify projectively who then become either friendly or hostile to them. They either fascinate or provoke rejection.

This is found especially in borderline patients who have a hysterical superstructure. The hysterical component makes it difficult for them to tolerate not being the center of attention. You may love them or hate them, as long as you notice them explicitly. Some narcissistic patients can behave in a cool, manipulative way. They attune the group to themselves and merge in it, even if it consists of only seven other patients and the therapist; they regard individuals as unimportant, and use the group as a single object with which to fantasize a symbiosis that affords narcissistic support.

Narcissistic patients may seem retiring and indifferent, cool and consciously manipulating, or markedly dogmatic. How their basic narcissism shows depends largely on other components of character. Thus dogmatic behavior is found particularly in narcissistic-compulsive patients. Depressive members have partly reached a depressive position but often have very serious problems of self-valuation, so that they are easily offended. The therapist should realize that narcissistic development may be viewed as an attempt at coping with a particularly frustrating environment.

Paranoid behavior is found particularly in patients who combine schizoid and compulsive traits. Some of them structure a group in such a way that it becomes the persecutor, in which they often show strong "interactional power" (König 1982). Others hide their paranoid fears by silence and confirm their expectations by selectively perceiving fellow members' behavior and by projective identifications. Depressive, easily offended patients rarely stay silent for long, because they have to produce concrete relations to objects; but they do keep quiet when offended, when they often are left to their self-hatred, even to the danger of suicide. Permanent silence can arise in depressive, "unwelcome" patients who feel superfluous everywhere. In the differential diagnosis of the various forms of silence, nonverbal behavior is vital. One can usually recognize whether a member is silent in a participating, defiant, offended, or paranoid-anxious manner, whether he feels welcome or superfluous, or whether, for example, he phobically avoids and fears to stand out in the group (König 1986b). If in doubt, one should address patients toward the end of a session, not only to wait and see if they may not talk after all, but also because some can say more about themselves if they know that the session will soon end, so that the fixed time frame would prevent them from becoming involved without limit.

Transferences codetermine whether a patient speaks or not. Some patients as children attracted attention by stubborn silence (Kreische 1986), when they were the odd one out in the family. Some patients predominantly experience their conduct in the group as rivalry with the father and want to avoid rivalry disputes (like some men who are hysterical or homosexual or both). Finally, there is transference of the guiding object (König 1986b), with aspects both of character and of transference: the need for a guiding object arises from deficient ego structure and from a wish for familiarity.

In general, a person's behavior depends much on character. Thus depressive patients can project their own impulses to exploit on the group, keeping silent because they feel speech to be verbal self-depletion or fear to be sucked dry if they show themselves to the group. They do this in all phases of group development, or only in those where other members' behavior offers appropriate transference triggers. Exploiting objects may then be transferred.

Patients who keep quiet because they are afraid to offend may behave like this mainly from characterological habit or mainly from motives of transference. Finally, some patients know that they can indeed offend, because some ego functions are not developed enough, or are paralyzed by conflict, especially as regards anticipation of how one's behavior affects others.

In terms of ego psychology, the development of character comes from a change of initial relational wishes through the action of defense mechanisms. The theory of object relations stresses the constant influence of inner objects on habitual human behavior: objects that are habitually transferred into relations, with the patient trying to reproduce his inner world externally, by selective perception and by the interactional part of transference. Doubtless the most effective procedure is to keep in view ego-psychological and object-related aspects of theory together or in turn, while noting what mobilizes defense mechanisms: whether they become active by habit or only if linked with certain sets of transferences.

Defense mechanisms involving retreat from self or external reality are a special case. In everyday life, they appear only in patients of very weak ego. In a healthy person they arise only from severe traumatic influences (Jacobson 1964). Patients in individual analysis speak mostly about such disturbing changes in their perception of self and others; in groups the same patients can be retiring and silent. Here details from the case history are useful if related to a patient's ego functioning. Being deprived of a clear sense of self and reality can be worrying indeed; moreover, the attendant distancing from bodily self and from the environment can prevent the patient from using the group process. However, this also serves as a protective mechanism. In our experience, such detachment in groups is mostly a defense against dangerous destructive impulses following frustration. Silence can show that the a patient's tolerance threshold has been crossed. Hardly anyone can from the start unreservedly face changes that therapy may cause in his view of himself. Having to face errors in this view can make one feel insecure and offended. In that case, one is less afraid of speaking than of hearing answers one expects from the group.

Patients unused to speaking are often afraid of ridicule. This is quite normal. However, someone with a phobia about blushing who fears he will blush when speaking shows a symptom of illness.

Problems about education and social class are involved in the fear not only of ridicule but also of not being understood. Besides, class is often put forward to rationalize oedipal fears of rivalry; here middle- or upper-class people supply triggers for the transference of parental objects.

Moreover, disowned exhibitionistic desires may be involved, especially phallic ones, castration fears, and the fear of one's own castrating tendencies along with the wish to keep the other intact; likewise the fear of revenge by the castrated victim.

Some patients find no intimacy in a group because they cannot lodge their transferences. The group does not provide transference triggers that create a family feeling for them and so they stay silent, sometimes in resignation or fear. If one addresses them on this, they often put forward external things, perhaps that members of the group have other interests or live in another world, and so on. Actually, the other group members provide no triggers for their transference needs.

As mentioned earlier, the therapist's task with silent patients is to frame hypotheses on their silence, and to decide whether to address them or not. Addressing them might consist of asking how the patient feels, of stating suppositions, and even of commenting on observed behavior. Asking is the gentlest method, because it is closest to social custom and leaves the patient the choice to reply or not as well as what to say. A supposition suggests something definite: if it applies, the patient may feel exposed; if it does not, he feels misunderstood.

The danger of provoking exposure likewise exists when nonverbal behavior is addressed. Here, too, it is expedient to abide by what is socially customary: it is best to address what is generally recognized as communicative, such as facial features and gestures. Posture of body or legs, often directly linked to sexual fantasies, should be addressed only if the working relations with the patient and between the patient and the other members of the group are relatively stable. Verbal interaction with a silent patient should not start with an intervention that might expose him.

Quite generally, one must watch how far a patient has developed a system of communication based on good working relations. A therapist who has not yet interacted with the silent patient but with the others has at least shown, by the way he dealt with them, how he works in the group. A patient can prevent the development of a working relation by differing totally from the therapist as to the proper course of the therapy. This happens especially with compulsive patients. If such persons fear expulsion when they show that they wish to work quite differently, this problem will remain untouched. Here we stress the importance of the preliminary talks, when the therapist should ask how the patient thinks the group can help him and how it might work. The therapist must carefully watch whether the patient seems to conceal objections.

The interactional routine of a contact-disturbed patient, for example, in the form of ironic provocation, brilliant intellectualizing, or self-mocking caricature, can turn out to be a recalcitrant resistance, since it is hard to get behind it to make disturbance manifest if the patient has no other ways of making contact. His solutions are mostly less than optimal, since his ability to interact is restrictive. In the end, questioning the patient is usually indicated, without completely condemning him. Sometimes it may be necessary to screen such resistive contact behavior from the criticism of other members by stating that it has advantages. Often the main thing is to widen the behavioral range rather than replacing it with a totally different one. Resistances impede other ways of seeing things. Psychotherapeutic jargon with which a patient has become acquainted may be used for this. Such a term is "performance pressure." A person disturbed in work may never have experienced that performance and need not always be motivated only externally. Depressive patients who lack drive find any action a burden, because they are motivated by calculations of expediency or by demands of the superego or ideal self, but not by the wish to work; phobic patients are frightened by any impulse to act; hence their reserve as regards the work in groups.

In every therapy there are demands on patients to perform. A patient has to work in order to progress. Some therapists, especially depressive ones, who are not rare, have a bad conscience when they expect patients to perform. They create the illusion that everything will run of itself, but secretly resent patients wishing to remain idle in the group and devalue them internally. Further, some of these therapists tend to ally themselves with subgroups that protest against performance, protecting them from others that like to be active and expect the same thing from the idlers. What he takes up or leaves alone in the group can likewise be linked with the therapist's structure. A schizoid therapist afraid of intimacy will encourage the group to aggressive discussions; a compulsive one provokes aggression and relishes it openly or in secret. Such conduct often has the result that spontaneous aggression cannot occur, since the therapist is obviously expecting it.

It is indeed easier for the therapist to control behavior than to discover that he is defending against impulses, for example, defensively muting aggression in favor of caring. Equally, rejected impulses of phallic rivalry can lead a therapist not to query a member who is after the therapist's role but even support him, although for that patient and often for the group as well it would be a drawback if the aspirant were succesful in rendering the therapist powerless or in inappropriately taking over some of his functions.

Some people are gifted in quickly reaching interpretations, but they still lack a vital skill of the therapist, namely, the ability accurately to foresee the effect of interventions and so to dose and time them correctly. If a member indulges in wild analyzing in the group, his behavior should be addressed, in his own and the others' interest.

In this connection let us point out that hypomanically repelled depression can mislead a therapist into inexpedient activity. Overcompensated primary contact disturbances in a schizoid therapist may lead to excessive and scaring offers of contact. The therapist will easily note whether he is devaluing members and can check this more readily than idealization that can overtax a patient or a group. A therapist inspired with a patient's abilities may lose sight of what is going awry in the patient's and the group's life. Such enthusing can be based on suppressed envy. Counterphobic analysts afraid of offending (König 1986b) can drive patients into foolhardy enterprises by acknowledging foolhardy plans of action. Hypomanic overoptimistic therapists, or hysterical ones with impaired powers of testing reality, can overestimate a patient's progress and so end a therapy too soon, as well as overrate his possibilities in private and professional life. Finally, a therapist conducting groups should reflect on his own situation in life, since his transference needs depend on how far his inner objects already correspond to external relations.

Even if a therapist makes an effort not to show his preferences and fears during therapy, he will not always succeed in this. Real-life solutions, such as separating conflictual relations or putting up with a hopeless relation, can influence his attitude toward his patients' relationships (see König and Kreische 1991). This holds for relations both within and outside the group. We must always remember that personality is formed not just during the first few years of life. The importance of adolescence is becoming increasingly recognized; later years are still being neglected, or considered only with regard to restaged oedipal conflicts, or at best adolescent ones. All adult conduct is indeed influenced by the past. However, relations with inner objects often admit several types of adult relations, and which is chosen may depend on chance. Once a person makes a choice and bases his future on it, he may find it hard to accept different solutions in others and to realistically assess their chances and drawbacks. Here the patients in a group can act as a good corrective.

König often tells his groups that all people are different: a truly trivial intervention, but one that often brings surprises. We all know the fact but not all have really acknowledged it. Intellectually many patients know that there are various solutions fitting different people variously. Still, many have a secret ideal notion how people should live and behave in certain situations. This clearly holds for compulsive patients, who must do everything "right" and therefore cling to their ideals, but also of schizoid ones, who have learned to deal only with those on the same wavelengths as themselves. They never got close enough to other kinds of people to appreciate that those had other ways of living. To such schizoid patients the group offers a good chance to broaden their attitudes and their scope for relations. With compulsive patients the fear of the "false" must mostly be worked on as an analysis of defense possibly hiding behind sham tolerance of what is different, often in the form of "What I tolerate may be all right in others, but I would never allow it in myself (hence I am a better person)."

Group therapists should not forget that the group is not the only important item in members' lives. Thus a member may be so excited by events in his outside relations that he continues attending to them within the group. He may be afraid of unpleasantness if he talks about them: he would be revealing himself through his outside relations and might incur criticism.

A patient might feel that his problem is out of place in the group for the moment. There are those who always think that their concerns are out of place. However, the other members may in fact be concentrating on forms of relation belonging to another phase of development than those that engage the patient now. His fear that what he wants to say would be ignored is then partly based on the actual stage of the group process. In twice weekly groups, patients tend to consider relations inside the group more than in less frequent ones. Hence in low-frequency groups more "individual therapy in the group" tends to occur than in groups of higher frequency. If Garland (1982) is right in that a group must essentially offer a system competing with those in which the patient normally lives, this effect will be stronger in twice weekly groups than in once weekly ones.

Initial silence of the whole group is to be distinguished from silence that arises during a session. The former is often necessary after long breaks, to enable members to become reacquainted, visually to start with, for example, on first meeting after a vacation by the therapist.

Preverbal fantasies are often conveyed nonverbally. Thus a group fantasy develops that would not have arisen had the patients spoken. When patients do begin to speak, it becomes clear that a group fantasy already exists, without anyone needing to have said anything. Protracted silence tends to raise members' anxiety, if they are able to feel it. Few of our groups have kept silent for over 25 minutes, but this seems to vary from therapist to therapist. The therapist's own nonverbal behavior certainly has an influence here.

Initial silence can, of course, turn into a sterile ritual. It can serve evasion: "Let others go first." Some groups, especially in an anal phase, will keep silent to show that they can tolerate it.

The therapist's nonverbal signals will partly hinge on how he perceives the silence, whether he feels at ease or whether he fears the silent group might escape his control, and on how he assesses non-verbal communication in the group. Some assume that nothing happens if nothing is said. Silence might mean that the group becomes depressed, growing ever less enterprising. Such silence should be addressed, since as a rule a group can hardly overcome oral regression unaided.

If the therapist is careful, he can usually recognize which patients wish to speak but dare not, which merely wait, and which become depressed. All this shows in nonverbal behavior.

Common silence unites and helps patients to focus on the group as a whole. In analytic groups silence can be left to go on longer than in psychoanalytically oriented ones. This follows from the level at which one intends to work. In the analytic group what mainly matters are collective group fantasies that arise in regression; the main concern is transference on the group as a whole and on the therapist. In analytically oriented groups one seeks to clarify the relational network in which the patients' inner conflicts operate (see Foulkes 1990a, 1990b). This is best achieved when unifying regression is low. In a psychoanalytic-interactional group long silence is not admitted, since early disturbed patients then become too anxious, and it is for them that the procedure is mainly designed. Their nonverbal communication is often disturbed or very selective in what they perceive.

What common group fantasy arises during silence depends on the state of development of the group, among other things. Fantasies related to the phase before triangulation ("dyadic fantasies"; see Ermann 1985; Rotmann 1978, 1985) are mostly directed to the group as a whole. The therapist is included or he is viewed as the group's protector. In oedipal fantasies he usually figures as an individual distinct from the transferred group. The role of the parent of opposite gender is taken on by individual members, more rarely by the group as a whole. Still, it may happen that no common unconscious fantasy arises. Everyone is "elsewhere." This may be a defense against wishes for amalgamation, by standing apart.

The safest move with a silent group, as with a silent individual, is to intervene by asking a question. The therapist might ask what sort of silence this was, and what mood was prevailing. Or he might confront the group with his own perception by saying that the silence seemed tense, or relaxed, or whatever. It does make a difference if he adds how he reacts to his perception, whether it makes him anxious or impatient, for example. This conveys an affective response, sometimes proper in psychoanalytic-interactional groups. The therapist should ask himself not only why he wants to intervene when he does but also why he remains silent when he does. His silence might be countertransferential rather than expedient; he may, for example, be afraid of separating himself from the maternal object, by stepping out of or standing out from the group. This occurs particularly often with therapists who like to intervene, saying "we" when "I" would be more correct. Or the therapist may pretend that it is not because of his position that members esteem what he says more than what the others say.

The therapist can drift into fantasy and feel paralyzed or anxious. He may remain silent because he is preparing "perfect interventions," or he may fear his interventions might not fit at all, especially if he is a beginner. Or he may be silent from almost any of the motives that also apply to patients. Therapeutic ideologies, too, may hamper the therapist. He may regard it as all-important that the group process should develop without directive intervention. He may radically reject the role of leader, because he has had bad experiences in leading roles or because he tends to direct and must keep this in check. He may ward off his own sadistic tendencies that might come out in interventions. His silence might indeed directly express sadistic impulses by consciously leaving his patients dangling.

Silence on the therapist's part is particularly unfavorable if a therapist's resistances creep in. It can be particularly harmful if by keeping silent he fails in his protective function, for example, if a patient is tackled in a wounding manner or if the group cannot cope with a monopolizing patient.

The tendency of a therapist to remain silent from fear can be warded off by an opposite tendency to be hyperactive, by interpreting contents or resistances too soon, or by relying on the traditional role of leader. Resistance can aim at maintaining an operative though suboptimal solution when better ones might be reached. To this extent the therapist maintains the principle that the better is the enemy of the good. However, a resistance may be as yet required to advance a group process (optimal level of resistance, see p. 68). Action is needed if members tend to skip their resistances instead of overcoming them. Silent groups that have discarded useful resistances are very hard to influence.

Chapter 15

Particularly Difficult Patients

One of the most difficult problems in a group is a patient who behaves in a very offensive manner. This is not always because such a patient is unable to foresee the effect of his behavior on others: the offense is often deliberate. The aim may be to devalue the other in order to be able to feel better oneself. At the root of this lies bad self-esteem. Sadistic motives are rather rare; when compulsive structures were more frequent one saw them more often. So-called castrating women are often taken to be motivated by penis envy. As shown in more detail elsewhere (König 1991b), this occurs when a girl has identified with her father because she related badly with her mother. There is then a discrepancy between a woman's anatomy and that of the object with which she identifies, so that she is constantly reminded that she cannot be like her father; a woman who has identified with her mother would not feel this envy except perhaps symbolically because of the advantages that men have in our society. This form of motivation is rarer than often assumed. Women with bad self-esteem often behave in a "castrating" manner because they are looking for the most vulnerable spot in a man, exploiting his fear of castration. This fear is particularly marked in phallic men, since they feel unsure of their maleness and therefore overstress male sexual attributes. There is such a thing as male "castrating" behavior toward women. It may be directed to the imagined phallus of the female, or to the sex characteristics making a female an attractive potential partner. The motives correspond to those of castrating women: a generally bad self-esteem or uncertainties as regards personal sexual features. Castrating behavior springs from doubts not only as to the person's own potency or physical attractiveness, but also as to charm and other personal assets.

The ambivalence of a woman to her own genitalia usually concerns identification: she experiences them negatively if she feels she ought to be a man. As direct opposites of female genitalia she imagines male ones. The attitude toward one's own body, for men as much as for women, often expresses itself in hygiene, dress, and so on. When a person in a group alters his mode of dress, the therapist needs to ask himself to whom this change is aimed: himself, the group as a whole, a subgroup, an individual patient, or someone outside the group. Sometimes new clothes show improvement in self-esteem; occasionally a decline in the latter first shows in neglect of appearance.

Some patients seek confirmation of their attractiveness by starting an intimate relation with a fellow patient. It is not uncommon for this to occur between a man and a woman, or between two women or two men if they meet often and exchange intimate details. This usually impairs therapy. The interaction of two such persons inside the group becomes minimal: their outside mode of conversing would not be fitting in the group. Each tries to give a favorable account of himself in the group, because the partner is present. Besides, anxiety about speaking of sexual fantasies in the group is heightened if the possibility of realizing them is shown. Some group therapists think that at least one of such a pair must leave the group if intimate relations arise. We hold that one should decide in the light of particular circumstances.

Patients usually know quite well that such relations are bad for therapy. They serve not only to confirm a person's own attractiveness. A male patient, for example, might wish to deprive the male therapist of a woman in the group, or a female patient a female therapist of a man. Idealizations might be involved; the relation with the group becomes more intense through an intimate relation with a member.

All motives based on transference, which might surely be further extended, result in the other being seen less realistically than if one had met in ordinary life. Thus a relation that arises in the group will be less successful in the long run unless the partners develop further in the course of therapy, each toward the object imagined by the other. Usually they force themselves to correspond to what is expected in the relation but cannot endure this for long (König and Kreische 1991).

Patients who monopolize a group by always moving to the center of events may have the most varied motives: phallic-exhibitionist, narcissist, phobic or counterphobic, masochistic or sadistic. Some sadistic patients monopolize in a way that makes it hard to protest, for they have become very skillful at lodging their sadism in relations. Often a monopolizer wants to control the group by star-shaped communication: everyone interacts with him. Some monopolizing patients induce a bad conscience in a member who fails to attend to them although they are unwell. Often a monopolizer suffers a lot. This cannot be permanently changed if he manages to force his style on the group. Some textbooks make suggestions on how to deal with monopolizers in general, but this seems unrealistic, for there is no uniform type. Monopolizing behavior is the common final stage of different internal processes that need to be diagnosed and clarified. A compulsive patient who wants to control the group must be handled differently from a counterphobic one who wants to prove to himself that he is courageous, or a phobic one who feels unprotected unless all others look at him. If the motive becomes clearer, one can usually handle monopolizing behavior quite well, but not always. Some people feel at ease only in a monopolizing stance and are afraid of any other form of communication. Here one may have to remove the patient from the group: neither he nor it can progress while such behavior lasts.

The situation is similar with the so-called help-rejecting complainer, who complains but will not accept help. If he stopped complaining, he thinks he would be giving up having relations with other members and feel abandoned, offended, devalued, deprived of influence and power, and be expelled. To reject help will maintain a special communicative structure: it must be rejected; otherwise the reasons for complaint might diminish or disappear. Perhaps, though, the patient has a different idea of help, for example, not through insight and new experience but through compensation, in that therapist and group supply now what the patient has missed in childhood.

Every therapy more or less has this function too. It is one of the secondary effects of psychoanalytic therapy, or it stands out in special measure, as is often the case in psychoanalytic-interactive therapy. However, this side of therapy can never work on its own, because patients expect to be compensated in excess of what is actually possible. Before compensation can be effective, such a patient must reduce his demands for it. That, however, frightens him, because he cannot imagine any other forms of help. Only in time will he grasp that there are other forms, by noticing what other patients are doing, what happens with them, and how they develop further. The problem, though, is that a group cannot be expected to be able to put up with such a patient long enough, as it can with a silent schizoid patient. Even if the therapist were equable enough and the members cooperative, therapy in the group would be much impeded by such conduct, because it constantly draws attention to itself and offers scant scope for therapeutic use. For such a patient to receive treatment he would have to drop his behavior.

Removing patients from a group is always awkward, because members develop guilt feelings that are hard to treat or they fear that if they become unpopular in the group they, too, will have to leave, or because the group as a whole would feel traumatized by the loss of a member. Help-rejecting complainers should therefore not be taken into group therapy in the first place. In individual therapy the therapist is better able to confront a patient with his behavior and to address his fears and suspicions, without his feeling exposed in front of others. However, he cannot then be shown by other patients of a group that there are other forms of object relation, which in turn restricts the prognosis.

Some group therapists tend to accept into a group patients whom they feel unable to treat in individual therapy. We strongly advise against this. Such patients often succeed in giving a group a dysfunctional structure and thus hinder the therapy of other patients as well. In deciding on an indication, one must recognize one's own limitations and those of a group. Therapeutic successes of psychotherapy are considerable compared with those in many other branches of medicine. However, among psychotherapists there seem to be many who find it much harder than doctors in other branches, such as internal medicine and neurology, to bear the fact that there are patients who cannot be helped, at least not with the means available in psychotherapy. This may lead to patients being deprived of drug therapies that might ease their condition. There are many reasons why psychoanalysis can be idealized; much of this is linked with the high commitment involved in becoming an expert. However, psychoanalysis alone is not always fit to help every person; sometimes drugs or even social psychiatry may be needed, as Kernberg allows and recommends (Kernberg et al. 1989). Choosing a therapy that is not really indicated can rest on ignorance and lack of skill; anyone can make a mistake. However, it often rests on unreflective illusions of omnipotence and sometimes it is an act of sadism.

Chapter 16

Preparation and Initiation of an Analytic Group Psychotherapy

PRELIMINARY TALKS

After conducting the preliminary psychoanalytic interview and taking the case history, the therapist formulates an indication. Let us assume it favors analytic group psychotherapy.

If a patient is not already keen on taking part in a group, having gone to the therapist with this aim, one usually must work out such a motivation, since most patients expect help from the therapist in the first place. If the therapist recommends individual therapy, the dyadic setting of preliminary talks gives him a chance to interact with the patient and so acquaint him with the psychoanalytic mode of working. At the same time a positive transference usually develops, motivating the patient to trust the analyst. The group therapist has the additional task of motivating the patient to work with other patients.

For group psychotherapy more than for individual psycho-therapy the patient can have only a limited notion of the procedure to be followed. Later, in the group, he will undergo experiences hard to foresee since in this shape he has not had them in other forms of groups, such as working groups. Besides, not only the quality but also the quantity of information needed for a complete picture would be larger in the group case than in the individual one, because group psychotherapy is more complex. Hence the layperson finds it more difficult to gain an overview of the attendant phenomena. If one wanted to tell a patient everything that might happen in a group, it would require study over a long period. Even so, the emotional aspects would be absent. Such detailed information would moreover have the drawback of inhibiting a patient's behavior, making it harder for him to profit from the group.

Still, the therapist should give some hints on how the patient can derive therapeutic use from what he will learn in the group. In patients who have interpersonal difficulties one can start from the symptoms complained of and point out that in the group one can enter relations without consequences in the world outside, clarify them, and gather new experiences in them. In patients with symptom neuroses in the strict sense, such as compulsion or anxiety neuroses or neurotic depressive disorders, interpersonal difficulties are often not spontane-ously admitted. Such patients should certainly be asked to describe themselves as persons, which usually reveals these difficulties. One can point out that intrapsychic and interpersonal difficulties are often connected. Most patients readily understand that interpersonal trou-bles have something to do with experiences in the primary family, and that these influence what adults expect from relations. With some patients it is enough to point out that the difficulties they mention are usually related to the symptoms: since they cause pain by themselves it is sensible to work on them. Such hints are recommended for patients who lack experience in drawing conclusions by analogy. If a patient obviously cannot draw them, this may counterindicate analytic psychotherapy, where such conclusions are central (König 1991b). Many patients are afraid that they might catch fellow members' symptoms by a kind of psychic infection and so become more ill than they are already. One can ask such patients whether they have prior experience of this. Usually one discovers interpersonal difficulties based on specific inner problems, for example, a restricted ability to delimit self from others in experiencing them (König 1991a). If this restriction is marked, one may have to revise the indication for analytic group psychotherapy. If it seems indicated nevertheless, the patient should be told that he has an interpersonal problem here that needs to be dealt with. The objection "why should sick people be able to help me?" may lead a therapist to fantasize with the patient how it would be if the group consisted only of healthy experts. Further procedure then depends on what fears and expectations this brings to light.

Another useful question: Does the patient trust himself to help others? One then learns something about how much psychic energy the patient can muster for working relations with other members. At times it is important to point out that in ordinary life the patient is surrounded not by experts but by others like himself who have more or less similar interpersonal problems. Along with this the therapist can state that the range from psychic health to psychic illness is continuous and that no one is ideally healthy.

Patients who raise many objections but at the same time seem strongly motivated for group psychotherapy should make the therapist reflect: maybe they wish to push him into the role of an over-careful parent who discusses all possibilities with the patient, as a mother would with a child going on a long trip when she thinks he cannot tackle possible difficulties. Excessive care and anxiety can be signals for trying to put a therapist into the role of a helping, ever-present, all-powerful, and all-foreseeing object. One can usually tell this apart from healthy skepticism. If the therapist tries to understand the patient in preliminary talks and shows that he is doing so by confronting and clarifying interventions, the relation that usually develops will be positive, as earlier mentioned, and the patient will feel understood. What is much more frightening than a refusal to satisfy drives, for a child as much as for a patient, is absence of understanding of his needs and wishes, irrespective of whether they are fulfilled or not.

If the patient feels that he is understood, he is usually ready to give the therapist the provisional trust mentioned earlier. Besides, a positive relation protects the patient during the first group sessions and makes it easier for him to identify with the working mode of the therapist.

The therapist should indirectly point to his protective function by asking what the patient might be particularly afraid of in a group, thus showing that the patient's difficulties in the group and his fears do interest him, too, and that he wants to take account of them.

A relation can develop in very little time. In some self-awareness groups, participants are accepted without prior interview usually without trouble, if they have some previous knowledge of psycho-therapy from what colleagues at the same or a higher level of training have told them about the theory and they have by then developed some personal relation and affinity for group psychotherapy. Such colleagues mostly succeed in transferring to the therapist and to the group the provisional trust, which shows itself in their choice of profession and place of training. Besides, colleagues can readily find out how competent the leader is. A patient is in a different position. What he finds out about the therapist is often vague and comes from other patients. Such information is often colored by transference, thus giving a limited view of the real therapist. Patients are also unfamiliar with the psychotherapists' professional group. That is another reason for having several preliminary talks with patients. As regards explicit information, the patient should agree. Implicit ones, as described in Chapter 10, at least facilitate his entry into group therapy. What is explicitly discussed beforehand seems to vary between therapists more than other things, especially as regards forfeits for missed sessions and the arrangements for vacations. Agreements must be adapted to the patient's situation and mutual as to financial risk: it should be made clear when the cost of a missed session falls on the patient and when on the therapist.

If patients are familiar with so-called body therapy, the difference between that and analytic psychotherapy must be discussed. In particular, patients given to aggressive outbursts had best be reminded that they must renounce any violent moves toward other members or the therapist.

Patients who have been in body therapy sometimes cannot see the point of refraining from bodily contact in analytic groups. Usually they will understand the explanation that in group psychotherapy the main issues are desires and needs that are at first unconscious because their possible fulfillment would provoke fear. By excluding actual fulfillment of aggressive or libidinous drives, such needs can more readily become conscious and accessible to treatment.

A further caveat for the therapist's inner attitude: In groups, transference brings out desires for relation whose fulfillment in childhood would have broken the taboo on incest. Usually such oedipal desires remain unfulfilled; if not, the consequences are traumatic. However, there is no point in explaining this to patients, for the account would be alien. For the rest, therapists fulfill many preoedipal needs of patients by focusing attention on them, understanding and holding them, feeding them words, and being reliable; but they do not fulfill oedipal-libidinous desires. Also, therapists let themselves be attacked verbally in groups and will tolerate much of the aggressive behavior that people in our culture commonly exhibit.

A therapist's clear inner position on the rule of abstinence matters especially because otherwise he may give his patients contradictory signals during preliminary talks: for example, if he has a bad conscience when imposing the rule or if he feels sadistic as a refuser of wishes. If his conduct in refusing is extreme, it may in fact be rooted in unconscious sadism of his own being defended against.

Recommendations regarding contacts outside group sessions cover a wide range. The site of sessions no doubt has some bearing on this—if you're in an anonymous city or in a small town where patients cannot easily avoid each other. In any case, outside contacts should be discussed during sessions.

Keeping to these rules, the point of which can be only in part explained to patients, requires some provisional trust and therefore a modicum of positive transference. Not that the relation to the therapist might not be ambivalent, but it should have a positive side. It may be enough if the patient hopes that the therapist can help him.

If during preliminary talks the relation goes from positive to negative, or the patient begins discussion with aggressive feelings and behavior that seem to rule the relational domain, the therapist must suspect an early disturbance with a strong tendency to split objects. It is then risky to rely on the patient developing a positive transference to the group as a whole, seeing that he rejects the therapist. Usually the patient develops negative expectations of relations with the group, too, and makes them come true by projective identifications. For example, he may behave provocatively, so that members actually reject him and he has to leave the group. Being intensely afraid of the group while idealizing the therapist may likewise point to object splitting.

The question of forfeits is somewhat topical. An empty place in the group cannot be filled; the 24-hour rule (the patient need not pay if he cancels attendance for a valid reason 24 hours before the session; what counts as a valid reason should be made quite explicit) thus will not mean what it does in individual therapy. Nonetheless many group psychotherapists use the rule to distribute risk. If the patient cancels by the rule, the therapist bears the financial loss, if at less than 24 hours' notice, he bears it himself. Such an arrangement is usually accepted because of its mutuality.

The therapist should be aware if he cannot convey this mutual aspect to the patient. Such patients might see the forfeit as a punishment, as if the agreement came not under civil but under criminal law. It takes time to treat the superego problem behind this, so that in preliminary talks the therapist in most cases can do no more than bring the confusion to the patient's notice. Clear rules on forfeits make later treatment easier, if conflicts arise in the course of growing transference and hook onto this question. It is often quite fruitful to treat such conflicts. They are often linked to ideas and expectations that are conflictual for the therapist himself. To test this in his own case, let the reader consider the following case: A patient for the first time in his life wants to go on an interesting trip or allow himself some other luxury, and at the same time wants the therapist to give him "leave" for the trip, although this goes against agreements.

The forfeit has another special position in therapy, because by withholding payment a patient can exert direct and real influence on the psychoanalyst. The latter does use the fee in his own daily life, outside the psychotherapeutic situation. The retained fee is like the opposite of a present from patient to therapist, which the patient expects the therapist to use in his daily life, outside sessions. Gifts and retained fees are counterimages of each other. Further, some group therapists are afraid to be accused of greed or pedantry in the bounded setting of the group if they insist on financial agreements.

EARLY SESSIONS

At the start of group psychotherapy, a double aspect of such an enterprise becomes particularly clear. On the one hand, the therapist sets up an experimental situation by not fulfilling the expectation conventionally directed at a group leader. Conventional adult behavior that has become habitual loses its grip in such situations: participants cannot rely on the leader leading in the conventional sense and then themselves behave in a complementary way. Motivated by instinctual desire, impulses to action arise, provoking fear and corresponding defenses that show themselves in therapy as resistance. The group as a whole, individual members, and the therapist in various combinations constitute transference triggers, and members try to satisfy their instinctual desires in relation to the transferred objects that they see in the others. Besides these desires, the wish for familiarity is important (König 1982, 1984), which contributes to the members trying to make other members' behavior resemble the earlier behavior of familiar objects, by transferential projective identification.

On the other hand, in group psychotherapy one is meant to work. What is to be worked on is experience and action in the quasi-experimental situation. This involves abilities both on the part of the therapist and of members, who cooperate with the therapist and with each other in working relations. To acquire these abilities one needs appropriate ego functions, which the therapist may temporarily take over, and there must be enough motivation to do the necessary work. The basic positive relation to the therapist, mentioned before, will make it easier to learn via identification. The teacher must ensure that the learner is stretched neither too little nor too much, and is given clear information. This means, among other things, that the leader must intervene intelligibly, above all in early sessions, in doses that patients can grasp and emotionally accept. Otherwise they experience failure and lose the will to work.

Clear interventions make apparent what the therapist is after. In supervision groups one observes time and again that from therapists who intervene clearly and in proper doses, members learn to deal concisely with essential matters in the spirit of the therapy. Resistances that occur will likewise be fairly concise. A therapist who knows how to orient himself in the group, giving apposite interventions at the right dosage, makes his future work in the group easier, since concise phenomena are easier to diagnose. The whole group process becomes more efficient. That members of groups where the therapist intervenes in this way can deal with essentials more directly depends also on the fact that an apposite interpretation makes patients feel safe, which reduces anxiety. They notice that the therapist understands them and recognizes their needs, even if he does not always satisfy these; they hope that he can protect them in difficult situations.

By taking on therapeutic skills, members develop their own feeling of competence, which enhances a feeling of their own value. Besides, they will find it easier to go on applying part of what they have learned to self-analysis.

In later sessions it is easier to take the risk that an intervention will be grasped by only one or a few members, or that it becomes clear only in the course of the group process. To avoid this in early sessions, interventions had best be such that presumably all members can grasp and emotionally assimilate them. Such interventions must not be too sweeping. In the first session more than later the danger is that the therapist overtaxes members with his interventions, not only because members do not yet know the requisite mode of working, but also because at first the anxiety level of a group is usually higher than later, and fear inhibits cognitive faculties. This fear is increased if members do not understand the therapist and therefore feel insecure. A vicious circle begins: members do not understand the therapist, become afraid, understand him even less, become more afraid, and so on.

Depending on patients' makeup and disposition to act, some individual members may then break off. A whole group breaks up more rarely, because there is usually some hope that things will improve.

If he behaves in an unusual way, the therapist should explain to the patients why. For example, it is unusual if he does not answer direct questions. He can for instance say: "Let me answer this later. What I find more important is why you asked this question." Thus he moreover doses the degree of lack of structure in a group, which he must adapt to the patients' tolerance thresholds. If an explanation is given and the same question recurs in a later session, it is advisable to confront the patients with the fact that they have heard an explanation and apparently forgotten it. Then the therapist should ask why this happened.

Frequently, patients try to "improve" structure. Taking turns is a favored move, each member for one session. This may be variously motivated; it can sometimes lead to analytic group psychotherapy being transformed into therapy of individuals with the help of a group. Since such structures lower the long-term efficiency of a group but will quickly establish themselves, they should be addressed in good time as being resistive, not omitting the protective function (which indeed exists in all resistances).

Information at the level of working relations has the secondary meaning of limiting the degree of lack of structure, by the therapist showing the patients how they are to deal with what they experience in the group and how they behave themselves. In this way the therapist gives implicit hints as to action. It is peculiar to group psychotherapy that even in early sessions deep regressions can arise. This is because the group as a whole acts as a trigger of early transferences and attendant ego regression. Further, this happens because patients, facing complex possibilities of relations with a whole range of people (at least some of the normal forms of conventional conduct being suspended), experience a feeling of helplessness related to that of very young children in a situation where their own actions cannot foreseeably meet their needs. Feeling helpless and dependent on a big mother object (the group) that behaves unpredictably would seem greatly to contribute to the development of transference forms that correspond to the state of development in the first year of life.

In the early sessions the therapist moves between two extremes: if he imposes too much structure, he deprives patients of the experience of early forms of relation in the therapeutic situation; if too little, the patients grow too anxious and their mental powers of digestion are overtaxed. The therapist should thus aim at structuring not to a "minimal," but to an optimal degree.

Because of anxiety that arises when patients have to face the unknown and experience deep regression with attendant feelings of being helpless and dependent, it is vital to monitor the balance between resistance and impulse. At the beginning of a group, the group process is most expeditious and intense, and the patients' gain in knowledge and experience greatest, if just so much impulse becomes manifest as to produce anxiety that would approach but not exceed their tolerance threshold. If impulses rise beyond a certain strength, resistance rises even more.

Alongside the structure introduced by the therapist, the forms of resistance introduced by the patients have less effect on feelings of fear, shame, and guilt. When a group begins, the patients know as yet few ways of dealing with their fears. In time, the available range of resistive forms widens. For that reason it is important not to activate the group's impulses too much; the unrefined psychosocial moves of defense early in a group may at times be insufficient, and patients retreat into the particular resistance of silence. This is rather difficult to deal with if the therapist so far knows little of the group and is therefore uncertain in judging it. The ability to regulate the level of resistance is one of his vital skills; members, too, acquire it with growing experience of group psychotherapy. When silence arises, the therapist must mention the protective character of it and relate it to the preceding interpretations that probably exceeded the patients' tolerance threshold. Or he may address the behavior of some members that had provoked fear. In this he should convey to members that he has recognized the rise in anxiety through the phenomena described and understands that they wish to protect themselves accordingly.

Careful dosing of interpretations of resistance and content early in groups is important because in the initial phase breaking off occurs more often than later and is particularly traumatizing at that stage. These are narcissist traumata, often fantasized as irreversible mutilations: the group has lost a vital part or organ, and so each member has as well, since what is fantasized is a symbiosis of mother and child.

If, in spite of precautions, a breaking off does occur, the therapist should tell the group that he has advised the patient concerned in a private discussion on further therapy. If the early sessions reveal that an indication was wrongly framed, for example, that a hysterical structure concealed a borderline structure that now shows itself in the group, it may be necessary to remove a patient early. This usually has an even more traumatic effect on the course of the group than if the patient breaks off. If indications are carefully made, the occurrence is, fortunately, rare. To limit the damage, the therapist had best make it clear to the group that he has made the decision about ending the therapy in the interest of the patient concerned and of the group. Even then members will have guilt feelings and fear that they might be expelled if they show themselves as they really are. Such feelings should be carefully dealt with and not denied in a collusion between group and therapist. The therapist's own guilt feelings are left to him for self-analysis. It is usually not advisable to burden the members with this.

In open-ended groups where vacancies are filled by new patients, each of the latter goes through his own initial phase. Depending on the stage of development and state of the group he will be seen as an unwelcome competitor for the therapist or for the group's attention, as savior and messiah, as close friend or partner of the therapist, and in many other roles.

As a rule, new members quickly adjust themselves to the stage of development of the group and then follow the group process of open-ended groups, cyclically repeating ever different stages of individual development. Still, the therapist, when framing his indication, should consider whether a given patient will be able to connect with members' unconscious fantasies in the current phase of group development or whether these happen to concern particularly explosive desires that the patient wards off. In that case, the patient might simply not understand what is going on in the group and block his experiencing, so that he will not learn how to communicate with the group in its own specific manner. This in turn bears on his further development in the group, if indeed he remains in it. Rationalizations, such as "all the members are married or unmarried or have a different profession, etc.," then often conceal the deeper problem. Such reasons may be relevant but are not always so. Some patients leave the group because they cannot lodge their transferences and therefore can develop no feelings of familiarity.

In most groups the newcomer is given time to find his way in. Established members expect some basic information from him, partly to create a minimum of trust. They allow him to remain reserved. He is then given a collective demonstration of how a group works.

Patients with a strong tendency to giving set views on matters that they do not yet know too well and of which they have little experience are more likely than others to find themselves in difficulties. Patients used to taking a leading role are more at risk than those who behave more like followers (gammas) in the sense of R. Schindler (1957/1958) and Heigl-Evers (1978).

Some patients who have learned only how to interact as scapegoat soon set up this (to them familiar) situation in the group. It is then important to show how far such a scapegoat represents latent desires of the group, and to find out what the patient himself contributes to this.

Patients who like to see themselves as expert advisers and enjoy this role are often tolerated for a fair period in this position if they are good at it, for example, if they do not create the impression of being omniscient but rather introduce new perspectives compatible with what the group has so far attained and with its mode of working. However, a parallel is drawn to the behavior of the therapist, who also holds back, and a conflict arises about the duty to take on the role of a patient.

Especially at risk in early sessions are patients with flimsy defenses, who soon say more about themselves than members are wont to or have learned to say, or want to hear. A cohesive group with some experience of therapy can usually limit or stop such patients; if not, the therapist must try to do so.

Chapter 17

On Ending a Group

THE END AS INTEGRAL PART OF THE
WHOLE THERAPEUTIC PROCESS

In a psychoanalytically conducted group, as in any therapy that aims to do justice to the reality principle, discussion of the nature of ending cannot be left until the concluding phase. Time and again, even before entering it, patients must deal with separation, farewell, and grief (see Lindner 1991b). A mother reports that her children are about to leave home; each year, during the summer months, there is quite a long break in the regular schedule of group sessions; a patient falls dangerously ill; a patient wants to stop treatment—the list of everyday triggers for remembering the end goes on. Such triggers force members individually and in common experience to consider the problem of termination. Depending on the individual and collective state of the development process, they will have to cope with matters like separation from the dyad of the early mother–child relation or later separation and threshold situations and the attendant feelings of pain and grief but also growth (Grotjahn 1979), with utopian fantasies and realistic possibilities, and, mainly implicitly, with the fact that one's life is finite. Dealing with the end is thus integral to psychoanalytic group therapy.

FACTORS DETERMINING THE END OF A THERAPY

A psychoanalytic group therapy occurs in a range of possibilities that is not unbounded, but under limiting conditions that help to influence its end. Three types of factors can be distinguished: the framework conditions, the patients' aims, and the therapist's aims.

Framework Conditions

It makes a good deal of difference whether the psychoanalytic group therapy is conducted in an inpatient or an outpatient setting. In the hospital one counts in weeks or months, as a rule from 4 weeks to 3 months. In outpatient therapy one counts in years, usually from 1 to 3 years. The length depends also on the times allowed by those who bear the bulk of the cost for group treatment in a hospital or in ambulant practice. Money is an ultimate factor, whether institutional or private funds. In the latter case the amount one can afford or want to allow for group therapy partly sets the time frame for the therapy. This hinges on how much a patient is willing to spend on therapy. Considering what people spend their money on, the usual fees for group psychotherapy seem not unreasonable in many cases. Many patients in psychoanalytic group therapy will have their fees paid for them.

Financial limits accorded in applications and requests for extension of payment have the effect of making patients see that time available for therapy is limited. Clearly, the topic of limitation crops up in various forms, for example, as limited lifetime, limited support for individuals and members as a whole, and will be the more incisive if time available is bounded rather than seemingly endless. From the start, this not only forces members not to lose sight of initial conscious and unconscious expectations, goals, and possibilities of development, but also triggers transferences.

The limitation of available time by those who bear the cost can split transference, so that the picture of the "bad mother" is projected on them and that of the "good mother" on the therapist. This can sometimes be encouraged by the therapist if he does not distinguish between his argued criticism of the grants and his therapeutic task in the group process. Criticism of the payer may be aimed at the therapist himself. Perhaps such criticism conceals an unconscious or preconscious pondering over the question whether the therapist provides adequate nourishment or whether he fails to do this.

If a therapist agrees with his patients that they themselves will pay after the grants run out, that transition can lead to inner debate in some patients triggering transferences reminiscent of adolescence. the time when one increasingly assumes responsibility for one's own life; however, regressive breakdowns may occur.

If these or other kinds of transference that can be triggered by the external framework are neglected, important conflicts will remain unattended.

Patients' Aims

The duration of a group therapy further depends on the expectations and conceived aims of the patients. One of them may wish to leave the group when his own expectations have been satisfied, another because the therapy disappoints him; a third will use the disappointment as an occasion for revising his initial expectations, conceive new aims, and continue. All this is found in comparative studies on psychotherapy. For example, it has been said that unfavorably developing psychotherapeutic processes and break-offs often arise from too low a measure of agreement between patient and therapist as to the conscious expectations from the treatment (see Fürstenau 1979).

The psychoanalyst must take an interest in patients' consciously and unconsciously conceived aims. In favorable cases, they will be mentioned even in the preliminary psychoanalytic examination and discussion, and at that stage bear on whether psychoanalytic group psychotherapy is indicated. Later they are the object of therapeutic work, though over long periods they will be dealt with indirectly. In the group-therapeutic process, which may be compared to the transference neurosis of individual analysis, it can happen that a member's unconscious expectations of himself and of the results of therapy, which are linked with the individual neurosis, are staged together with the other members and can then be worked through. Viewed in this way, a therapeutic process in the group is a digesting of partly unconsciously determined expectations of oneself and of therapeutic possibilities. Such a process opens new avenues of development by forcing the patient to give up expectations and wishful fantasies that could never come true.

In so-called balance sheet sessions, perhaps at the start of a new year, but above all in the final phase, the past work in common will be assessed, and it is a vital part of the therapeutic task to further this. Some therapists hold regular balance sheet talks, mostly in an individual setting.

Therapists' Aims

The problem of idealized normative aims as to ending psychoanalytic treatment has been worked out by Eva Stolzenberg (1986). Such conceptions may find expression in two ways: either by starting from ideal notions of aims about abilities that should be developed in psychoanalytic treatment, or by thinking in psychoanalytic terms and setting a certain stage of development of psychosexual maturity as an ideal target or norm and measuring the actual attainment against it. Whether this is perceived or expressed in more phenomenological terms or in strictly psychoanalytic ones, such targets can cause the therapist difficulties of countertransference as to daily therapeutic realities and of argumentation; for now the patients' actual reach of development must be justified in terms of an ideal norm, which can lead to a concealment of facts. Ideal normative aims can quickly turn into guiding images (and often tyrannical authorities) to which patients must become equal. This, too, shows how difficult it is to discuss the topic of limitation freely and openly. Every psychoanalytic treatment, even if optimal for the patient concerned, is limited in at least two ways: by the individual scope for development in each person and by the therapist–patient relation in which development occurs.

To take account of this, the therapist must know his aims and learn to deal with them. A discussion of these aims follows.

A therapist cannot rely on intuition (Glover 1955) to know when a patient has adequately profited from therapy and when to end it; then the results of therapeutic work would remain largely uncheckable. Intuition and feeling have their part, but assessing therapeutic progress also concerns the rational evaluation of countertransferential feelings and fantasies. The analyst is somewhat like a dowser, but he disposes also of geological and chemical gear.

Intuition and feeling, along with reason, belong together like conceived aims and the testing of them. The psychoanalyst reflecting on the end of treatment faces a task similar to that of his patients. He, too, must become clear as to his own unconscious expectations from therapy, including his own skills, his ideas of the therapeutic process and of his patients' scope for growth, his conscious aims and actual progress in development, but also the regress of members; first intuitively, then in a more rational way. Unconsciously determined expectations in the form of countertransferential feelings and fantasies will be discussed elsewhere. Here we deal with conscious ideas of aims only.

Since the first now classical formulations by Freud (1914, 1928) of the aims of psychoanalytic treatment, later authors have modified them to suit their own theories. Two basic notions remain the same: a patient should recuperate his ability to perform and enjoy, and the ego must grow where the id ruled. These aims cannot be reached in all therapies. Besides, one cannot describe health in static terms, but only dynamically (Ticho 1971). Moreover, Freud's theories make clear that discussion of the aims of psychoanalytic treatment is from the start determined by the tension between abstract arguments in formal metapsychological terms and material ones in everyday language. Value notions of the therapist enter as well. In psychoanalysis the mention of therapeutic aims confronts the patient with this tension. One cannot put oneself outside it. That this is true of Freud himself is well known. It was shown by Scharfenberg (1968) from where Freud's everyday formulations of ability to enjoy and perform might derive: from Sephardic tradition. Metapsychologically put, a group therapist, to judge therapeutic progress in his patients, must keep in view their development as to ego, instinct–ego-ideal, and superego. Let us try to put this in concrete terms.

In general, then, therapeutic progress shows in the way relations develop, of patients relating to themselves and others, to work, play, and other sublimations, and to objects and ideas (Menninger and Holzman 1958). Better relations to oneself, for example, a more conciliatory attitude to oneself, can be tested in certain aspects in the psychoanalytic sense.

Viewed from the aspect of ego development, at the end of a treatment there should be no further splits between regressive and actively controlling sides of the personality. A patient should have become more self-perceptive and better able to bear personal discomfort. The ego-ideal and superego usually develop following culturally conveyed guiding pictures and standards (Menninger and Holzman 1958). This also reveals how far a person has gone in dealing with the gap between narcissistic fantasies and real possibilities.

Changes in the superego are usually taken by psychoanalysts as the most important indicator of successful therapy. From this point of view, a good therapy will enable a patient, who started with a cruel, unpredictable, or crudely bribable superego, to have a freer and more enjoyable life, and compulsive activities and depressions will diminish. The content of valuations and therefore of the superego will change. A person who, for example, "loved" work, money, home, and power, may become more aware that these were compensations for human relations.

Time and again one finds patients who first learn from others that therapy has changed them. Thus therapeutic progress shows up in relations with other people. Often it is through psychoanalytic therapy that a person first discovers another person as such, and can give up a narcissistic spin and the satisfaction of infantile desires in favor of maturer relations and possibilities of satisfaction. For example, the patient need no longer compete with his children or with child symbols for satisfaction of infantile, pregenital desires. Moreover, one expects that therapy will develop of greater stability of objects and of gender identity.

Relations to work, play, and other sublimations and to things and ideas will change during therapy, so that, for instance, the interest in work will rise, as well as the attendant satisfaction. People with blocked creative powers may discover them for the first time. One who used work as a substitute for relations will find that this no longer satisfies. One who earlier lacked interest in play may now discover it. If play was overcompensation or substitute satisfaction, it will now lose importance.

This attempt at specifying concrete aims of psychoanalytic therapy could be continued. In sum, the therapist must be clear what the possibilities for each particular patient are.

Therapeutic processes in psychoanalytic groups traverse phases that can be described in terms of psychosexual development (König 1976). These phases are different in closed and in open-ended groups (in the latter, members enter and leave). Group therapists must understand that not all patients in a group are engaged equally strongly in all phases. Open-ended groups show clearly that patients can profit from a group without having taken part in all phases that it may have traversed in the course of years.

We thus once more stress the variable possibilities of development and limitations of patients. In recapitulating the aims of psychoanalytic therapy as regards its use in groups, we have seen the tension that has always existed between idealist-normative aims and realistic ones that consider the actual set of relations and possibilities of development.

ENDING IN DIFFERENT SETTINGS

What has been described so far has a different impact depending on whether the group is closed in an inpatient setting, closed in an outpatient setting, or open-ended in ambulant practice.

Closed Groups in an Inpatient Setting

These are defined by the common start and end of therapy and constant membership. If no member leaves or enters and the duration of therapy is fixed, the therapeutic process can develop undisturbed over a long time. Since a common ending of the therapeutic work is expected, it contributes to an intense and lasting experience of the common farewell. Members must separate not only from each other and the therapist, but also from the community that no longer exists after the last session. This fact usually triggers specific transferences to the group as a whole. It awakens memories of experiences with the early mother, who goes away and perhaps will not come back. Depending on whether the leader is male or female, the content of unconscious fantasies will differ. A woman leader may run the danger of no longer being seen as distinct from the group as a whole, so that working separation through becomes even more difficult.

Termination of closed groups in a hospital involves farewell from the clinic as an institution, where patients have "alighted," often for several months, into a protected space of a common life. This encourages regression to farewells experienced in early childhood or adolescence, in the family or in such groups as kindergarten and school. Moreover, having thus assembled in a safer place from most varied backgrounds usually entails intense work on each patient's return into the rough outside world. We hear repeatedly that the joint farewell of a closed group in a clinic is among the most intense experiences of leaving and crossing thresholds one can have, similar to the collective farewell and the pursuit of a new path in life on leaving school.

Closed Groups in an Outpatient Setting

Sessions are not as frequent as in an inpatient setting (3–5 times weekly). They occur usually once a week, sometimes twice. Also, there is no common experience of a clinical institution. This makes farewell and threshold experiences less intense than in an inpatient setting. For the rest, the fact of a common farewell acts in a similar way and shapes the common process.

A therapist who wants to work with closed groups in ambulant practice must decide whether financial providers or other institutional conditions set the time frame, whether he himself will have to set overruns, or whether agreement as to ending therapy is to be left to the process. Each variant involves its own considerations.

The End of Therapy for the Individual in Open-ended Groups

Open-ended groups are marked by the replacement of those who leave. Changes should not occur too often, because constant departure and arrival are not favorable to analytic work. Still, that members leave and new ones come is not merely a tribute to reality. It favors certain experiences represented in the here and now of the process in open-ended groups, if indeed that is not the only place where they occur. To be a newcomer in an alien group is such an experience, which not by accident has been pointed out by Jewish colleagues. To have been new and alien has been not only an important topic in Jewish history since the exodus from Egypt, but often the personal fate of these colleagues (Lindner 1990b).

Here, too, the setting shapes the process, sets transference triggers, and calls forth specific resistances. It almost goes without saying that those who take part in open-ended groups more often face topics like "every person needs his individual time for development," "birth," "leaving the parental home," "substitutes," "loss," "being a newcomer," "xenophobia," "death," and other factors, depending on the setting alone.

An experience can be put to therapeutic work in this way only in open-ended groups: if a member leaves, he must face the fact that therapeutic sessions will go on afterwards since the group continues. This fact will become a trigger and actualize hitherto unconscious conflicts, for example, envy of those who are nourished at home, safe and shielded. In this sense open-ended groups are closer to the ones in which we live as adults.

TECHNICAL QUESTIONS

The End as Topic of Preparation

The end of a psychoanalytic group treatment should be a topic even in the preparatory period for group therapy. In general, patients' expectations and questions of finance give them a chance to speak of the length and term of therapy. If the time of ending is not fixed from the beginning, the therapist can point out in the preliminary talks that this hinges on a process of agreement in the group, in which evasive moves and other forms of resistance may be expected.

For open-ended groups we suggest that in preliminary talks an agreement be struck with patients that a wish to end should be announced, at least 3 months before the intended end, so that sufficient time is left to work through leave taking. Mentioning duration and end in preliminary talks has the advantage that limitation of the available time has been mentioned from the start, even if the attendant problems can be treated only in the course of therapy.

Pain of Separation and Experience of Growth

If members wish to end therapy together or if a member leaves a group, not only the actual farewell but also past experience of leave taking is revived, even if this has already been the subject of earlier therapeutic work. As in individual analysis, in the final phase of a group increased regression, livelier transferences on the therapist and on the group as a whole, and a return of symptoms may arise, as if the unconscious were protesting against the decision of the ego (Menninger and Holzman 1958). To digest the pain of separation, mourning time and energy are needed, as a group therapist is often able to observe from his countertransference feelings.

As mentioned before, the therapist must reflect that a farewell can be the start of something new and so be an experience of growth. If we remember that farewell as separation is not only a "little death" but also usually the start of independence, the therapeutic work will involve, along with pain of separation and mourning, joy in the new and the future.

Working on Resistances

Not every wish for ending therapy expresses resistance. Still, it is surely right to think in the first place that a resistance is coinvolved if the wish to end therapy becomes vocal. In groups such utterances always trigger events that soon make it clear what part resistance plays. In open-ended groups, individual patients often show resistance by stating, with all kinds of plausible reasons, a wish to end treatment just when discussion is about to turn to a topic that for them is full of conflict (see Lindner 1991b).

A typical phenomenon of groups resisting the disappearance of individuals is this: the majority holds on to the one who wishes to leave and attacks him fiercely because of his intention to leave. Often this goes with the fantasy that a member leaving would maim the group as a whole.

Resistance against ending therapy can include the therapist. In that case, all those involved unite in ignoring time. Given the constant presence of every resistance individually uttered, and of the formation of compromises involving everyone, the rule of thumb equating a wish for ending therapy primarily with resistance is plausible and useful. Of course, any therapy ends in resistance in the sense that the ever-present residue of pathological dynamics could be worked on further. Resistance helps the patient find the end when right for him, given his total life situation.

Countertransference

Here we will mention a few typical unconsciously determined problems of countertransference. (This is not the place for a general account of how countertransference must be handled, even in the final phase, or for the therapist's responses accessible to himself.)

Ticho (1971) cites one such problem, which he thinks many therapists have: "Some analysts are disappointed by the outcome of their training analysis. This more or less conscious dissatisfaction leads them to aim at 'perfect' results with their patients" (p. 45). Sometimes this goes with a kind of "researcher's jealousy," a fear of letting colleagues look at the therapy concerned. Perfectionist demands by compulsive therapists can lead to patients being kept in treatment longer than is sensible for them. Often this goes with a lack of confidence that patients will develop after treatment ends, when they shape their own lives and should go on working on themselves without the therapist's supervision. Compulsive and phobic therapists share such suspicions, the former fearing the patient might cause chaos, the latter that patients themselves will come to harm.

Conversely, hysterical therapists who desire quick results fail to see that a patient may not yet be ready to fend for himself; this is blotted out, because they wish to keep the illusion of quick results. Similar behavior occurs in phobic therapists who had distant mothers (König 1986b), requiring them to develop without help. However, if they want to proceed differently from their own mothers, they may keep patients too long.

Schizoid therapists overrate the effects of a patient's deep inner experience on his real handling of tasks in daily life; they underrate the need of working through the experience in detail. Obviously, a depressive therapist hangs on to his patients because he fears the loss of any object. Similar behavior may occur in a narcissistic therapist who views patients as extensions of himself, not as independent persons but as having important functions for him, like an arm or a leg. Such character features of a therapist may indeed surface in a closed group, too, when it ends as a whole. Therapists of any structure, who transfer a mother object onto the group, can behave toward the group as toward that object, which can be experienced as providing food and care, shelter and protection, supervision or guidance, and much else. Therapists can experience group members or the group as a whole as a child on the point of leaving them. Such a child may then be restrained or sent out from home too early; the latter partly in order to fulfill tasks and realize life chances that were denied to the therapist in his own history.

The reaction of a therapist to separation from a group naturally depends on his current object relations (König 1991b). Here the vital point is what place the group or its individual members occupy in the field of these relations. Desires for object relations that are satisfied by relations outside the group bear on relations to group and members less than others. Therapists without family will wish for different object relations than ones whose wishes are largely fulfilled by their family. Therapists who are acknowledged from several directions will feel less dependent on a group as regards acknowledgment unless they are insatiable for it. Finally, it is important whether the place that a group or individual members leave free in the therapist's field of object relations can soon be reoccupied or not. This may matter particularly toward the end of a therapist's professional career.

When a Whole Group Ceases

A therapist working with a closed group who does not set their duration from the start should keep apart two aspects connected with their ending: finding and fixing the end, and working on the farewell. Discussion about the time to end serves therapy because it tends to intensify the process. What is involved is not only farewell, separation, mourning, and revision of initial fantasies, but also such anxiety- and envy-ridden topics as comparing therapeutic results or the question about contacts after group therapy. For this phase a therapist should take sufficient time, given the explosive nature of the discussions that arise.

If a term to therapy is found by the group, and accepted by the therapist, it should be maintained even if suddenly some members question it, from fear of separation or for other inner reasons. Discussion on the accepted end should become central to therapeutic effort; revising it would encourage manipulative behavior in the group. Kadis and colleagues (1963) point out that the prospective end of closed groups can for some patients be an additional motive for getting well, but in others evoke a paralyzing effect. Such paralyzing phenomena point to strong basic impulses of destruction and aggression, which should be addressed, even if in some cases the therapist may feel bound to advise further treatment in another group.

When Individual Patients Leave

Quite often, patients start talking about the end of their therapy without this leading them into the final phase. In the attendant discussion it will become clear that certain conflicts and resistances lead to the threat of a break. Distinguishing between finding and fixing an end and the final phase is meaningful in altered form in open-ended groups as well. If one or more members wish to leave, finding and fixing the end and working on the farewell are not the same as when everyone leaves. In an open-ended group some want to stay and others to go, a tension in which the therapeutic process develops. A member's wishes to end therapy are best dealt with in the group, not in an individual discussion, which would sever the group's dynamics. Here one must take account not only of possible resistances in the would-be leaver but also in those left behind who oppose his leaving.

In open-ended groups, too, one should stick to an end once adopted. If a group stops collectively or if some leave, the therapist must face the well-known question whether in the final phase he is to become more active and personally visible. In that phase a main problem is whether transferences, particularly on the therapist and the group as a whole, are dissolved and both targets appear as what they are. It may make therapeutic sense, for example, to take up and confirm apposite perceptions about the real person of the therapist. Still, patients should be able to keep the therapist as an inner analyzing object.

There are indeed therapists who fail to do justice to the analytic task in the end phase because through sham professional behavior they try to forestall the analysis of reactions of disappointment, sometimes from fear that such reactions might signify failure in their work (see Ticho 1971).

Balance Sheet Talks

Some therapists offer such talks to patients, to be held several months after the therapy. Lindner usually recommends an interval of 6 months. In many cases a therapist could thus observe which intensive and productive postanalysis processes are worked through by patients independently. Most patients accept the offer. This was found by Kreische (personal communication) in a study of records.

FAILURES

Patients Treated without Success

In time, any group therapist will meet patients who regularly come to group sessions but in the end do not greatly change. However carefully an indication is formulated, it can happen, as in other therapies, that we can find out only in the course of therapeutic work how weak the ego is or how impervious is a person's character structure (Menninger and Holzman 1958). In such cases, it seems important for the therapist not to deny, repress, or rationalize feeling helpless and powerless because of a wrong indication. Besides, the therapist is thus close to the patient's problem in that he begins to grasp why defense and

resistance have to be so rigid. He may simply have to end the therapy
at a time that is least hurtful, and to discuss with the patient what
other therapeutic possibilities might exist.

Breaking Off

Some researches (reference in Yalom 1974) show that breaking off
occurs most often within the twenty first sessions. Between the
twentieth and fiftieth session extremely few patients withdraw.
Anyone who stays for at least fifty sessions will very likely improve.
Yalom regards 35 percent of dropouts in the first twelve to twenty
sessions as usual. Only after twenty sessions, he says, does a group set
and patients will genuinely commit themselves for a long period.

Reasons for breaking off can be varied. The therapist may have
made wrong indications, but it may not emerge until the first sessions
that the patient could not take the opportunity the therapist, though
aware of the danger of withdrawal, had offered him. Patients tending
to narcissistic retreat or to frequent denial of their touchiness often
tend to break off as well. However, the therapist himself may have
made technical mistakes. If so, the best provision for the future is a
confidential talk with a colleague.

A good way to diminish withdrawals, other than care in indication, are preparatory talks in which the therapist can consider with
the patient how it will be in the group. This can make patient and
therapist aware of possible neuralgic points, as well as making clear
that group therapy involves possible offense and phases of hard
disputation. Such talks will strengthen rather than weaken confidence
in the therapist. The authors of this book have withdrawal rates of
under 5 percent. We take this to be the result of careful preparation of
patients for their groups, with special attention to developing a
working relationship.

Patients with tendencies toward breaking off therapy or actual
withdrawals can cause a therapist some disquiet, ranging from a
feeling of isolation and feeling that everything is crumbling away
to panic countertransferential behavior. A therapist may then be

tempted to exert pressure on candidates for withdrawal. This, however, only accentuates their tendency to break off. In such situations, it is useful to remember that breaking off is often a restaging of internalizing modes of behavior, by means of which a person may want to conquer the other and realize his own will (Lindner 1991b).

With growing experience one will accept that some breaks are unavoidable because one cannot always avoid mistakes in indication; unforeseeable circumstances can trigger withdrawal, as do certain group constellations. Grotjahn (1979) points out that there are negative countertransference reactions that produce breaks. He describes five cases in which the therapist responded to hostile transferences with openly negative countertransferential feelings. The patients he describes seem to have had much early disturbance, which emerges as hostility to fend off closeness and as tendencies to split, degrade, and avenge.

INTERRUPTION OF GROUP TREATMENT

Some group therapists advise patients who have not adequately profited from being in a group, either closed or open-ended, to regard the ending merely as an interruption. This is indeed how the ending of psychoanalytic group therapy is usually viewed in a hospital (Kadis et al. 1963). Here, too, it is prudent to hold balance sheet talks that at the same time plan the future.

There are also specific indications for interrupting a therapy, for example, in cases of sudden massive regressions in the course of a group, triggered by acute and difficult circumstances and having led to severe ego collapse. One may then consider individual sessions alongside group therapy.

SUBSEQUENT DEVELOPMENTS

A group therapist should not forget that after the therapy has ended there are further possibilities of development for the patients on their own. In the first place, the so-called postanalytic process that has to be worked through independently belongs to any ending of therapy; in the second place, for anybody there are in life impulses that can produce change. It is hoped that patients will be able to apply afterwards what they have learned in the psychoanalytic process to solving their own problems (see Lindner 1981, 1982). The goal of unending analysis would thus be attained.

Chapter 18

Inpatient Psychotherapy from the Group Perspective

THE SETTING

Patients in a ward form a group, open-ended or closed: some hospitals, especially in universities with many outpatients, select from them a group of patients at one time who will also end their therapy together. At this stage a preliminary selection is made from diagnosed patients, which thus decides the composition of the group in the ward. If the number of beds is small, it would otherwise be difficult to gather groups that do justice to the therapeutic needs of individual patients; if there are more beds, this will become more possible. In such settings the indication for a particular therapy is often made only after admission. In a ward specializing in treating neurotic and psychosomatic disorders, all patients take part in a ward group; otherwise an individual therapeutic program is worked out for each patient, which will combine individual therapy, group therapy beyond the ward, nonverbal procedures, such as movement and formation, and even treatment by hydrotherapy. Patients from several wards are collected into groups that can be run on different lines.

A ward group should follow a single approach that suits all patients there. A ward where diagnostic pictures vary often has patients for whom an analytic procedure that mobilizes unconscious conflicts cannot be used at all or only after a long preparatory period; a ward group is therefore usually run according to group notions that focus on treating conscious and preconscious conflicts, thus supporting rather than destabilizing the ego. To these procedures belong the psychoanalytic-interactional form of the Göttingen model and the so-called theme-centered interaction (Cohn 1984), an interactional group procedure in which a theme is given, either by the patients or by the therapist. Core aspects of psychoanalytic procedure are here formalized. The so-called rule of priority of disturbance corresponds to the rule of psychoanalytic treatment: resistance before content. The so-called chairman rule, that everyone be his own chairman, corresponds to the implicit injunction in psychoanalytic procedure, that a patient should take the initiative and not wait until he is asked to speak. This implies the further rule valid for any therapeutic group: one speaker at a time, speaking to all. Since this is basically a formalized psychoanalytic procedure, though largely doing without interpretations (somewhat like psychoanalytic-interactional group therapy) and leaving unconscious conflicts more or less unmobilized, it is compatible with psychoanalytic procedures and can prepare for them.

The two procedures are similar in many points in clinical practice (though less so in theoretical terms). Moreover, theme-centered interaction is suitable for patients who in terms of background are not accustomed to take the initiative in a group discussion; they have not learned it in parties, unions, or associations.

Both forms help to build up ego structures, in that they facilitate social learning. Many impulses provoke fear (and so must remain unconscious) because they were not socialized, on account of early blockage. In the course of his development, the patient has not learned to transform impulses into adequate social action corresponding to chronological age. If the blockage were suddenly removed, the behavior produced would be infantile, which would be dangerous because an adult has the force and scope of an adult. It is one thing if a child hits out in anger, but quite another if an adult does. Using others and the therapist as a model, patients learn in interactional groups to deal with their instinctive drives in socially acceptable ways. If in analytic therapy a blockage from earlier times is dissolved, the impulses will meet possibilities of realization that have already been practiced, which can make for easier therapy (König 1991b).

Analytic or analytically oriented groups in a hospital run much as in outpatient practice. However, one can offer more sessions per week, because in a hospital setting the problem of finding suitable times for all is smaller or absent. Besides, patients there are not burdened with current tasks in a job or in a family and can therefore give all their strength to therapy. Further, in a hospital setting it is easier to catch phenomena of decompensation that can arise if conflicts are mobilized. The maximal frequency of sessions in a hospital seems to be three times 1½ hours or five times 1 hour; at four times 1½ hours, we begin to notice signs of overdosing (reinforced symptoms, new symptoms). Therapy in a ward combines various possibilities of therapeutic influence, as is well known: preliminary talks and case history, in which therapy is already being prepared; clinical visits; ward groups; other therapeutic moves, both verbal and nonverbal (the latter to be conceptualized in psychoanalytic terms). A vital factor influencing motivation in new patients is meeting others who are already in therapy. This is an argument in favor of admitting patients at different times. If patients are taken in together and have not been prepared as outpatients beforehand, much time is lost in the ward with motivation, because the therapeutic team is not backed by patients already in treatment. Besides, life in common in a ward is a psychosocial training field, where fellow patients address many conscious and preconscious psychodynamic aspects of individuals (König 1991b).

Transition from therapy in a ward, with its many offers and prestructured possibilities of contact, to outpatient therapy is not easy. It requires a change of attitude if a patient has to cope with the tasks of his work and family, attending a group once or twice a week, and no longer being in a structured setting, free from such tasks and provided with a greater range of therapeutic offers. The patient exports from the hospital the task of having to put into practice outside those experiences and insights gained inside, in a social setting, which, as a rule, is less indulgent and more opposed to open speech. If, in addition, a patient then has to find a place where he can continue treatment, he may well feel overtaxed. Many hospitals try to counteract this by giving the patient leave to seek such a place and to use his visits home for applying at least some of his new experience and insights, namely, that part which concerns the family, while experimental work during inpatient treatment will do the same for the workplace. Such attempts are usually not possible in the patient's regular job during inpatient treatment, but this has advantages, too. The patient will feel freer to try new ways of relating to his superiors and colleagues.

In large hospitals with long periods of treatment group therapy is conducted in closed groups. For shorter stays and in smaller hospitals this can often not be done. Such groups are then not slow open but fast open. This creates technical problems that influence the themes of group discussions, because the group has constantly to deal with new and leaving members (Lindner 1990a).

The task of inpatient therapy is often to win patients over. Those who would not otherwise find their way to a psychotherapist or for whom psychotherapy is not suitable to start with can find their way into therapy in a hospital and can then be taken into outpatient treatment. Still, it is remarkable how much can be achieved in a short time in a hospital with its wide therapeutic range. Since psychotherapeutic processes consume much time, most patients need further treatment. One cannot speed up such processes at will, but in a hospital setting they are widened; here the various group offers play a vital role. In a psychotherapeutic ward, but also and especially in hospitals where there are both neurotic and psychotic patients, it is essential to observe the so-called dynamic of the ward with its partly unconscious processes; from diagnostic evaluations so obtained one must draw the therapeutic consequences, which may not always consist of interpreting but also of taking organizational measures. Therapeutic wards may be so organized as to encourage regression, or as to limit it.

The therapeutic team's ideology regarding treatment will bear on the ward, indirectly and directly, because it influences the attitude of team members to their work and to the patients, and thereby their therapeutic actions. It is therefore important to find out how much responsibility for the patients' lives is in fact taken over by the team and how much should be taken over in terms of the team's ideology.

Among the hardest tasks of a therapist is a meaningful limitation of therapeutic contact. In badly trained teams it often happens that therapists proceed either by a rigid scheme or work as much as they can and not as much as would be expedient. This leads to time pressures, made worse because badly trained therapists tend to congregate in less desirable clinics. One thing that makes a hospital less attractive is often an unfavorable ratio of therapeutic staff to beds.

If staff members misapply and waste energy, and concentrate on those patients who are loudest and most insistent in their demands, one can try to compensate for lack of personnel by providing more group offers. However, if the therapists are badly trained, they often fail to limit regression in the groups, so that groups promote regression and intensify patients' desires for contact and caring while paralyzing their scope for taking over a part of the therapy themselves. This damages the reputation of group procedures.

Many of those who run psychiatric hospitals are not adequately informed about the vital role of further training in a psychotherapeutic clinic, and the time needed for a therapeutic team to discuss difficult patients; if this is neglected, it means more work in the end. If a team is badly led or badly trained, it will tend to shun patients in favor of team discussions, dealing more with each other than with the patients entrusted to them. This is diametrically opposed to conduct that is concerned only with the patients and neglects communication in the team, because the time spent on that would deprive the patient. Both extremes often have the same causes; they are inexpedient attempts at solving problems arising from these causes: bad training, defective structure, and excess workload because of a bad staff/patient ratio.

Often outside supervisors are asked to resolve conflicts in a team. This may be expedient, but the leader should be involved, if only because the result may require a change in structure. Otherwise there will be tension between leader and collaborators: the leader does not know why such a change was suggested, and his teammates underrate the time needed to catch up on what a team has gained under supervision (König 1991b). Suggestions for structural change are not always realistically grounded. They arise not only from rational reflection but also from conscious, preconscious and unconscious emotional needs, to be noted but not allowed to be decisive. A supervisor should not limit himself to a psychoanalytic view, but must take into account social and psychological aspects as well and have some notions on organizational structures if he is to work effectively; otherwise he leads the team into unrealistic actions, or he works only on the effects of inexpedient structures. This amounts to a kind of symptomatic therapy of the team itself, which is highly convenient for the administration of a hospital but not very expedient, at least not in the medium and long term (see also Fürstenau 1979).

Experience in using group models that include sociopsychological aspects (e.g., the Göttingen model and Foulkes's model) is a better basis for a team supervisor than models that neglect them.

PECULIARITIES OF SMALL GROUP TECHNIQUE IN A HOSPITAL

In a hospital there are exceptions from the phased run of closed groups. Having observed about twenty groups a year over 10 years in the analytic control seminar of the neurosis clinic at Tiefenbrunn near Göttingen, we have gained the impression that groups of short duration consisting mainly of schizoid and depressive patients sometimes fail to reach the anal and phallic phases. On the other hand, therapists who are against the short-term aspect of clinical psycho-therapy tend to arrest their groups in the oral phase by developing a dispensing conduct above all toward the group's oral desires. The result is that oral frustrations will not settle adequately and thus escape treatment; the therapists in question are mostly depressive types.

That a therapist drives his group ahead at high speed will not in general cause it to run more quickly through the developmental phases mentioned; rather, resistances grow stronger and the group will become fixed at one stage. The developmental phases will be traversed if a group is heterogeneous as to the patients' structures and the therapist does not block the main determining factor of this course, namely, the time limit, because of countertransferential difficulties that lead him to restrain or spur on the group. In a hospital setting it may be best to involve group members less than in ambulant practice regarding analysis of resistance. In the latter one is better able to wait until resistive behavior of individuals becomes clear to the others who then address it. Groups where the therapist allows greater indepen-dence find it easier in our experience to integrate newcomers than groups in which the therapist largely reserves the treatment of resis-tance for himself. In a group lasting only 8 weeks one has less time to wait. Integration of newcomers is, of course, absent from closed groups.

CHANGE OF THERAPIST DURING THE RUN OF A GROUP

In ambulant practice sessions will usually stop while the therapist is on vacation or has to absent himself for professional reasons, such as further training, or if he falls ill.

In a hospital one must consider the limited time a patient remains; leaving aside costs, patients are often prevented, by reasons of family or work, from extending their time for the length of the therapist's absence. When illness or further training keeps the therapist away, he must arrange for a substitute, even when he goes on vacation. Be aware that cotherapy for training purposes does not always solve the problem, if the more experienced therapist is absent.

A change of therapist naturally changes the course of the group in ways depending on the developmental phase, which includes current transferences and transference triggers, such as the gender and age of therapist and substitute.

That a change of therapist is not always unfavorable is doubtless linked with the patients who are staying on, besides developing transferences to the therapist as a person and as representing the hospital as mother (or father). Still, in the initial phase one had best avoid a change of therapist, for here the reliability of early object relations is at stake.

Example: After the third session, a woman therapist had to seek a substitute for 10 days. She had mentioned this in preliminary talks. During the first sessions, members avoided entering an emotional relation with her, leaving her outside, since she was soon leaving anyway. The substitute was a man with whom members did not want to relate either. After the original therapist returned she was still left outside, while members' utterances, which turned on bad parents, revealed lethal aggressivity based on disappointment. This was hard to handle for two reasons: she was on the outside, being ignored, without any working relation between group and therapist as a basis for communication; and she, who in analytic terms saw the aggression as aimed at herself, developed some corresponding countertransferences and became aggressive toward the group, which showed in her posture and facial expression. In a control session, the situation was clarified and technical means found to overcome it in part, but not quite. The therapist had as good as confirmed that "mother is not reliable," for she had left, and her time away was experienced in primary process unconscious fantasies as lasting much longer, feared perhaps as forever.

If a group has become convinced that the therapist is reliable (that he will always be there) to the extent that it can protest against dependence on him, it will be better able to digest a change of therapist. Stubbornly insisting that "we can do without him, namely, with the substitute alone," has a different meaning. In the oedipal phase of a group, too, a change of therapist is followed by reactions that are easier to treat than those in the initial phase, especially if therapist and substitute are of the opposite sex. The group's reactions correspond to those of children in similar situations in the family. On the whole, members in the oedipal phase, corresponding to the three-sided situation of the Oedipus complex, feel dependent not exclusively on a single reference person. As might be expected, the difficulties in this phase are greatest when a therapist falls ill, for in that case not only does the substitute enter the group unprepared by his predecessor, but also his falling ill seems to realize oedipal death wishes, which provoke guilt feelings. A change of therapist toward the end of a group is easier to deal with than earlier on, since by then members have built up a stable working relation with the therapist, who on that basis can give reasons why he has to absent himself, though his leaving will still influence the dynamics of transference in the group.

For patients with addictive problems, a change of therapist is a trigger situation that might lead to a relapse, a circumstance not always adequately taken into account. For such patients it is particularly important that a change of therapist is avoided or that these patients are thoroughly prepared for the change (Lindner 1991b).

Chapter 19

Indications:
Which Patient
into Which Group?

Indications for psychoanalytic therapy, individual or in groups, overlap. Not a few patients could be treated in either, though it is hard to give a percentage, since in both cases the range of indication depends on the therapist's personal style, as will have emerged at many points in this book. A long-term psychoanalytic procedure is indicated if the symptoms rest on a broad structural basis. If the part of ego pathology is high, one must consider whether the ego is strong enough to bear additional tension, which is sometimes, though not always, provoked by an unconscious conflict hitherto warded off becoming conscious and therefore directly active in the ego, when hitherto it may have shown up merely as a symptom that in the sense of primary illness gain relieved the ego. In some patients, especially with borderline pathology, the immature ego expresses itself directly in the symptoms. This must be taken into account in therapy, by taking over auxiliary ego functions in a wider sense than it usually occurs in therapy anyway, with a therapist, as it were, thinking and fantasizing ahead of the patient.

Group therapy above all suits patients whose inner conflicts express themselves in interpersonal conflicts but is also suitable for treatment of psychoneuroses where this is, or seems to be, not so. It further suits patients afraid of dyadic relations. Analytic group therapy, in contrast with long-term treatment, may help patients whose symptoms cannot be influenced, at any rate not durably, without changes in structure, but who at the same time cannot easily bear deep regression if it lasts too long. Deep regression in a group arises quickly, because the group as a whole is a powerful trigger of transferences to early objects. It also can more quickly be reversed than in individual therapy, because at the end of a session the group as a transference trigger dissolves into individuals, while in classical analysis the therapist, invisible during the session, induces regression that develops over a period and can last to a greater degree between sessions. Since in groups it is usually more difficult than in individual therapy to keep an overview of the current life situation of a patient, outpatient group therapy is on that ground alone less suitable for highly disturbed patients. In a group session of 100 minutes with nine patients, each gets an average 11 minutes, so that merely in terms of time it would be difficult to keep the therapist up-to-date on everything therapeutically relevant that occurs outside. In a group, therapy occurs through the group process, in which all partake at the same time, but less time is available for each member to speak, so that each can convey less than in individual therapy of 100 or even only 50 minutes a week.

Changing from interpretation to direction, as demanded by Kernberg (1975), if a crisis supervenes, is harder to implement in a group because directive behavior has an effect on the group as a whole, altering the therapeutic process not only for the person just involved but for all. If one had eight or nine borderline patients in a group, the therapist would spend much time on crisis intervention, at the expense of medium- and long-term therapy. However, it is quite possible to have one or two borderline patients in an outpatient analytic group, partly because the healthier patients take over auxiliary ego functions, so that, given relative numbers, crises are easier to master without detriment to the therapy of the other members. Borderline patients can help a group process because they are closer to the primary process than neurotic patients. Their function in the group resembles that of psychoneurotic patients in groups of psychosomatic patients: they present fantasies more remote from reality and more intense feelings. In regression a group always meets, as it were, an ego-disturbed patient who behaves and experiences in the same way as a regressed one. Even so the therapist must watch that such borderline patients do not act out destructively. If this tends to exhibit as violence or suicide or an addiction (alcohol, drugs, gambling), the patients should not be treated in the same outpatient group as other patients. Such patient groups must be homogeneous as to disease, because a certain behavior, such as drinking or gambling, is often discussed there, and no patient who conceals a relapse can claim as an excuse that a mention of it would have been unfitting in the group. Patients with strong suicidal tendencies in general should not be treated in groups, at least not without a tight-meshed individual therapy alongside.

On the whole, acting-out patients are more readily treated in ward groups, since the hospital setting offers a protective framework and a group is not the only opportunity for talking about acting out. Besides, acting out in a hospital is usually noticed by other members of the therapeutic personnel. Therapeutic visits and individual talks provide further safety. In a ward therapy the number of early disturbed patients in an analytic group can be increased. Still, in our experience this should not exceed three in a group of eight, and four in one of nine.

Psychoanalytic-interactional groups offer good scope for ego development and, even more than analytic groups, are a field for social practicing in which foreseeing one's own effect on others can be developed as an important ego function. The extra social skills gained present possibilities for dealing with impulses that can later enter the ego, during analysis of defenses in a psychoanalytic therapy. In any case, indication for group therapy in a ward is not the same as in outpatient practice, where no other concurrent therapy is provided (see Lindner 1989). That a patient has group experience from a hospital is not to say an outpatient group would be good for him. Since in a psychoanalytic-interactional group the therapist supplies much structuring and speaks on his own initiative to individuals more often than is usual in an analytic group, the patient needs less prior experience of groups here than in the analytic case to become involved in conversation at all. The counterindication against group therapy where group experience is lacking (Heigl 1987) holds mainly for analytic and analytically oriented therapy, but less so for psychoanalytic interactional therapy (König 1994).

Kernberg (1975) has shown that psychotic patients who lack sufficient discrimination between images of self and objects will get worse if one uses interpretations, whereas with borderline patients they can help. If a prepsychotic schizoid patient is able to keep quiet or at least reserved for a long time in a group, he can often take vital steps toward discriminating these images, since in a group the other members are more openly different and thus more marked than in everyday life. The prepsychotic patient can gain experiences that would not be possible there, if only because he mostly finds no contact with people whom he experiences as different, not on the same wavelength, if indeed he is not in any case debarred from close contact because of primary generalized contact disturbance. He can also correct transferences of immature inner objects, which are already separate from the self.

Schizoid patients who do not hold back on contact and borderline patients with general ego weakness often benefit from psychoanalytic-interactional therapy; likewise for psychosomatic patients with inadequate discrimination of affects. In the latter case studies of so-called alexithymia (Ahrens 1987) have shown how much apparent inability to experience and convey feelings depends on the situation. Clinical experience confirms this: many psychosomatic patients do not discuss feelings with a doctor only because they were never given an opportunity to do so (König 1979). Doctors who consider only the body are indeed often fearful of anything except physical illness and show that they want to hear none of it.

The effects of primary contact disturbance too can be somewhat improved in a psychoanalytic group where patients can watch others interacting and then begin to interact themselves. In the protective shell of a clinical ward essential progress can often be made; likewise for patients in a daytime clinic. In connection with outpatient settings, we earlier mentioned that for strongly acting-out patients groups homogeneous as to illness are the most favorable. That certain forms of acting are regularly discussed makes up for the drawbacks of homogeneous composition, for example, the overlap of blind spots. In assessing whether a homogeneous group is indicated, one must remember that not all patients with a certain diagnosis, for example, alcoholics, are equally strongly and similarly disturbed, and that there is hardly a specific alcoholic personality. One must distinguish between phobics who sedate themselves with alcohol, depressives who derive impulse and euphoria from alcohol, schizoids who use alcohol as a stimulus protection, and compulsives who are troubled by their conscience like depressives but want to be rid of their tiring efforts at control (König 1991b, Lindner 1987b). In bulimia, too, eating behavior rests on most varied conflicts, while the clinical picture of anorexia seems to be more uniform.

When planning treatment the therapist must be aware that patients with defective discrimination of feelings often do not know how to terminate unpleasant emotional states, because an undifferentiated affect gives no specific instruction on how to act, except to use a drug (König 1991b). Preconditions for adequate social dealing with impulses should be set up within the therapeutic framework. Psychoanalytic-interactional therapy here coincides in many points with behavior therapy (see also Heigl-Evers and Heigl 1983).

The psychoanalytically oriented form of the Göttingen model suits above all patients who will presumably get sufficiently well in a short therapeutic process (1 to maximally 2 years). Patients of high structural level with conflicts that are near the surface and therefore easy to treat are rare, and in such a process there is no time for broad treatment of all derived conflicts and not merely of their general structural basis. It is therefore particularly important in such a group that the therapist dig out, in individual sessions before the group begins, acute conflicts relevant to the symptoms, far enough to know them and draw the patient's attention to them. In this connection it is worth mentioning that couples therapy can produce such focusing. In the Göttingen department for clinical group psychotherapy six to twelve couples sessions come first and group therapy follows at one session a week for 9 to 18 months (Kreische 1986). The prior focusing seems to improve results in such a relatively short therapy. In Kreische's model therapy concentrates on the conflicts relevant to disturbances in the couple relation. In an analytic group psychotherapy, one often works on the plane of psychosocial compromise formation, on which one tries to concentrate, as far as possible, the therapeutic process in psychoanalytically oriented groups. There is, however, the additional possibility of allowing regression and even to promote it, in order to influence conflicts at the base of derived conflicts. In psychoanalytically oriented therapy, one indirectly encompasses the original primary conflicts, because derived conflicts share certain basic structures with deeper lying conflicts. In addressing the surface, one may include depths as well. In regression depths rise to the surface and can be worked on directly; basic conflicts thus come to the surface and become interpersonal, as happens for derived conflicts without regression.

Analytic groups where deep regression is used presuppose some ego strength in most members, since if a group not only has several early disturbed members close to primary process but also as a whole enters such a state, experience can be reflective only if members can leave regression as soon as the triggers that promote it no longer exist or are dissolved, by interpretation, for example. Regression here should serve the ego (Kris 1936).

Variants of internal conflicts that show up as interpersonal in daily life need more working through than ones that become so only in the group. In a group kept on the plane of mature compromise formation, the same number of sessions leaves more time for dealing with the interpersonal derivatives of earlier conflict; working at this level is suitable for dealing with character neuroses insofar as these are not among early disturbances with a weak ego. In such patients ego functions are often not undeveloped but only paralyzed by conflicts and hence "atrophied," whereas in early disturbed patients they are more often undeveloped.

It is particularly important in differential indication for group therapy to be clear whether ego functions are paralyzed, atrophied, or undeveloped: if paralyzed, one thinks of work with much regression; if atrophied, as can happen in progressed character neuroses, of work with less regression; if undeveloped, of a psychoanalytic-interactional group therapy. This last produces the preconditions for repression and the separation of ego, id, and superego or ego ideal, with corresponding defense barriers as required in daily life. Such a therapy can later be followed by analytic treatment.

If we speak of analytic, psychoanalytically oriented, and psychoanalytic-interactional group therapy here, this does not always mean that patients must be taken into a group run on just one of these models (see Lindner 1989). We have mentioned more than once that in an analytic group one can work on several planes. This is confirmed not only by the theoretical point that answer and interpretation are on a continuous range (see p. 73), but also the fact that in every analytic group there are elements of a psychoanalytic-interactional group, namely, in patients dealing with each other and talking openly about themselves and their relations to other members. Any group procedure that attracts members' attention to their mutual relations contains these elements in the foreground of the psychoanalytic interactional group. The therapist in an analytic group, in contrast to the psychoanalytic-interactional mode, keeps himself free as a screen for projections by saying little of himself. In analytic groups he can do this because members with more mature egos take on more auxiliary ego functions and can make healthier offers of relations than patients in a psychoanalytic-interactional group with often severe disturbances of the ego. There, the therapist has to be the prototype for perception and feeling, for the way of making contact and limiting it. All this may be superfluous in an analytic group with perhaps two early-disturbed members; here the other patients will do this. What a therapist behaving fairly naturally will reveal about himself in an analytic group is, as a rule, enough to maintain a personal relation with members on which to base therapeutic work.

Former inpatients who have undergone only psychoanalytic-interactional therapy can carry on in homogeneous groups, for example, in outpatient treatment centers for addicts. Why such groups are better for this has been explained earlier. As a rule, discharged patients who are severely disturbed had rather opt for an individual therapy, perhaps later complemented by group therapy.

As blind enthusiasm for groups has diminished and assessment of their therapeutic scope has become more realistic, we have become more cautious as to results to be expected (see König 1991a, Lindner 1991a). In group therapy, as in any therapeutic procedure, the more ill a patient, the slower his progress and the smaller the results. A healthier patient, in order to progress, can engage more ego functions from the start. This is shown not only by the Menninger project, which lies some time back, but also by more recent research (e.g., Luborsky et al. 1980).

An important indication for analytic group psychotherapy is the fact that regression can be experienced so as to lead to the underlying conflicts but will quickly fade at the end of the session, as discussed earlier (see p. 44).

Finally, frequency of sessions has a bearing on indication. More acting out can be dealt with if the group meets twice a week than if acting-out patients are seen only once a week. In the former case there is more time to discuss actual events outside the group, without patients' mutual relations (therapeutically the main feature) becoming subordinate. However, it is often hard to fix twice weekly sessions for a whole group of people. Besides, health-insured patients are limited as to claims. In a twice weekly group the therapist will much more rarely feel the need to see a patient in individual sessions and patients more rarely ask for emergency sessions. Third-party providers of funds would probably be well advised to raise the limits to claims for group psychotherapy. This might improve results and be cheaper in the long run (see Lindner 1990a).

A patient's age, too, bears on the indication for group therapy, as indeed for any psychotherapy. The older a person, the firmer the social bonds to which he is tied, so that putting his life and experience until now in question can produce fears that assume threatening proportions. Even if alternative lifestyles were available, a change of conditions can mean that a person will store up guilt toward others whose lives have become tied to his, for example, if he leaves them and turns to other people with whom he might be better able to live. The readiness to run risks (König 1974a) diminishes with the social ties that are entered in the course of life. Still, some become free again with advancing age, when children leave home. From self-awareness groups with older colleagues we know that in his mid-50s and even after 60 a person may still change. However, the therapist must take social bonds into account.

In groups, older members often fall into the position of parents to younger ones, because age itself offers the relevant transference triggers; if they themselves behave in childlike or adolescent ways, their "children" in the group become restless. Younger members often find it hard to accept that older people, too, can have childlike streaks and might wish to reveal them, for example, an infantile dependence on the group as a whole or on the therapist. Sexual desires and fantasies of older members strongly disturb younger members, for they arouse incest fantasies. The incest taboo being stronger toward the mother than toward the father, sexual desires of older women are more strongly taboo than those of older men (see Grotjahn 1983). Moreover, sexual desires of older women can no longer be justified in terms of possible reproduction (see König and Kreische 1991).

It is almost self-evident that in opting for group therapy, one must consider what kind of group is available, yet this is often neglected. Since the world over twice as many women than men ask for psychotherapy, the indication for men is often framed more widely than expedient for an effective, well-selected therapy. It is better to work with groups in which men are in the minority and to direct those men for whom this would be more suitable to individual therapy. A neurotic issue of the Oedipus complex with phallic identification in a woman who related badly with her mother and identified strongly with her father, and passive homosexual submission of men to their father, often lead to women being more active in therapeutic groups and to this extent resemble the male stereotype more than men.

As male and female roles in our society become more alike, this problem becomes minor, because gentle behavior in men and active behavior in women have become more acceptable. In so far as phallic overcompensation goes with devaluation of the "female" part of one's own personality, it can be useful for women to experience gentle behavior in men; but at first they may despise it, just as passive homosexual men may be afraid of "male-aggressive" behavior in women because they have to ward off corresponding impulses in themselves. The unfavorable effects of being in a minority in the group, mentioned by Heigl (1987), are now less important because sexual and ethnic minorities in society are more readily accepted, or at least it is agreed by the majority that they should be. Thus there are rarely problems with individual homosexual men, even if repressed homosexuality becomes active in the other men in the group. Homosexual women never had much difficulties in therapeutic groups. The growing spread of AIDS raises special problems in assessing male homosexuality; however, our admittedly rather limited experience suggests that they can be overcome.

It is becoming increasingly rare to find people who have no experience of groups, no doubt because of the greater number of residential communities and the spread of working groups in offices, factories, and schools.

Chapter 20

Group Psychotherapy
and Group Dynamics

In a therapy group members wish to diminish the displeasure caused them by conflicts and symptoms and to seek sources of pleasure so far denied them. In group-dynamic events members wish to learn to do their work better and so gain pleasure in functioning. In addition, they wish to work with less anxiety, which diminishes pleasure.

Group leaders and members thus pursue goals. Those of the therapist may have to do with his own advantage: pleasure in functioning, earning money, gaining experience, and so on. Participants pay him for promoting their goals. The participants' goals need not coincide with the therapist's aim. Thus a patient may merely wish to be rid of his symptoms, while the therapist in addition aims at a restructuring of personality. Correspondingly, the participant in group-dynamic training may aim at learning social techniques in order to apply them in practice, while the trainer hopes that in the course of the training the participant will learn techniques that will improve his dealing with people as partners. In either case the patients' or clients' value systems differ from the therapist's or trainer's; the leader hopes that the participant will adopt the leader's value system (if the participant thinks about it at all, though all this is often fairly unreflective). In some cases therapy is not begun because the gap between patients' and therapist's value systems seems unbridgeable. Greenson (1967) mentions this in his textbook on psychoanalysis.

If the gap must be taken as unbridgeable, therapists or trainers will often start working all the same, although participants have not given specific approval that fully respects the leader's aims. Besides, the leader's value system may change during therapy. We all learn from our patients or clients.

The demand that at the end of his treatment each member should clearly see the why and wherefore of the leader's conduct and have critically discerned the latter's value system is an ideal that points a way but can never be fully realized, at best perhaps in long-term self-awareness groups. Group-dynamic training is usually too short for this.

Psychoanalytically oriented group-dynamic trainers, whose goal is perhaps to improve participants' ability to cooperate, will above all address those aspects of the group process that impede members' mutual cooperation. The working relation itself will become the central object to be influenced, and its improvement will be the main therapeutic goal. In the stricter sense of therapy, too, it will be the goal, but not in the main. There it helps in working on conflicts that show up on the transferential level. A member who has learned in his group to develop better working relations will be able to cooperate better outside, too. This is one result among others in analytic group psychotherapy.

Further elements shared by group psychotherapy and group dynamics are that the group therapist makes use of regression, since it makes accessible to the group process otherwise hidden facets of personality. Group-dynamic trainers deal with regression, too. It helps them to loosen habitual behavior patterns and let them recede in favor of practicing new modes of behavior. Like the therapist, the group-dynamic trainer ultimately wants the individual to behave in a way mainly determined by secondary processes. If participants in a group-dynamic event work together at other times, too, that will limit the scope for individual self-awareness. The group leader must consider this.

Chapter 21

Groups with Physically Ill Patients and Medical Personnel

The task of a psychoanalyst working with groups of physically ill patients in many ways resembles that of a group dynamicist of psychoanalytic orientation. He should treat obstacles to the performance of the specific task of expediently dealing with limitations imposed by physical illness, just as a group-dynamic trainer wants to create the inner preconditions for tasks in professional life being solved better, more easily, and more satisfyingly. With the chronically ill it is not only a matter of better compliance with medical advice, which often entails limitations, such as keeping a diet, or effort, such as sports for coronary cases, but also inner processes of adaptation, such as from the identity of the healthy to that of the ill, who still want to live as well as may be (Biskup 1991).

The physically ill often deny their illness, and the possible later consequences, and the psychoanalyst must decide whether or not to address these denials. Quality of life can sometimes be saved only by denial. Witness the way each of us comes to terms with his own mortality—it is expedient to not *always* think of it. Many young people often live as though life would never end. They know that it will end, but they do not build this certainty into it. Older people, too, often try to live as though their lives were endless. If confronted with the ineluctable end, they start to consider life after death, be they religious or not. A nonreligious person will at least try to take care that his name will not be forgotten, and consider if and how he can live on in others or in his own deeds. He tries to order his affairs, to smooth the way for those close to him and sometimes make things more meaningful for them, to the best of his ability and understanding, by more strongly aiming at transmitting his own norms and achievements. In this task he often fails, and rightly so: in general, children and grandchildren must find their own sense in life.

Sometimes the fantasies of the chronically or fatally ill concerning their impending fate are worse than reality. They feel themselves at the mercy of those who have taken responsibility for them, which they gratefully accept, since it relieves them of responsibility. However, they might see those who try to help as best and honestly as they can as persecuting or senselessly restricting them. Not all who deal with the seriously ill will give all the attention possible, since they mostly have young dependents. These often represent more hope than the ill: most of us find it easier to bestow effort on those with a long future ahead of them than on those about to go. Being faced with imminent death and the dying of the chronically or fatally ill is for many bearable only within limits. One cuts oneself from the pain of others to protect oneself from being overburdened through identification with the afflicted. Team supervisors of personnel in wards with serious cases have to deal with such cutting off, but also with doubts whether enough has been done and with acknowledging their own lack of power, which often hides behind taking hectic but pointless medical measures.

One is constantly amazed how callously those who must tell the ill of their fate take the easiest way: complete and absolute openness, which replaces considerate and humane behavior. If psychoanalysis has an ideology it is enlightenment. In dealing with the chronically and fatally ill, love of truth can become cruelty if it deprives the patient of all hope, even if that would have to be illusory. If in Christian usage one says that everything will turn out well, this does not mean that one will be saved a serious fate, but rather that this fate can and will be mastered; witness the thought that a person must not go to ruin even when dying (see Koch 1989).

Healthy people who work with the chronically ill at times feel like psychotherapists who work in prisons. They are free of illness and of the need to come to terms with imminent death. They fear the envy of the ill, in whose place they do not want to be. Some treat the ill like weak children but at the same time overtax them beyond this state, because the attendants find their work more bearable if a patient is deemed to have much greater scope to develop and learn how to deal with his illness. However, in the role of child the patient may be disenfranchised by having everything taken over from him, being trusted much too little or not at all, just as parents can ask too much or too little from children. They constantly retreat to the position of the expert or of science, which is best able to state how to deal with illness, even if it cannot empathize with the ill. Medical regulations that make sense for younger or healthier patients, but not for old or ill ones, are carried through; a patient of 80 with a heart condition for whom eating represents an essential quality of life, for example, will be given a low cholesterol diet, though this can now hardly improve his arteriosclerosis.

Some doctors and nursing staff use such vetos in order to convey to patients that they matter. This is an unsuitable way to communicate, just as when parents who have no time for their children, or feel unable to provide the emotional attention needed for their welfare, have a bad conscience and spoil the children with material things.

A further problem is the impatience of the young with the old and ill, who cannot move or comprehend as fast as the young. The old become confused if forced to attend to several things at once, which a younger person can readily sort out and settle. The old must often be given information in small doses. Still, some old people feel underextended and offended if thus treated. Depending on primary personality, the old and ill try to make themselves popular with the nursing staff, or to gain attention by nagging criticism. Further, coping with age and illness depends on existing relations. Often the nursing staff has to stand in as the children, not only if there are none but also when they show little concern. It is often frightening how little children are prepared to care for parents in illness and old age, although one can understand it, because attending to the old and ill in a small family is not preplanned and can present insuperable problems. It would mean changing the whole style and mode of life. One often observes nursing staff being indignant at the children's lack of care for parents. Sometimes this is due to inadequate understanding, of the children's position as well: one does not wish to be like them on any account.

Personnel in intensive care units often come to develop an elite feeling, connected with mastery over complex apparatus, the putting up with burdens, and the power over patients, whose vital functions lie in the hands of the clinical staff. This attitude one should not question lightly. Often it is the one thing that makes the work bearable.

Perhaps more than in dealing with neurotics, questions of dosing are vital in dealing with the chronically ill and with medical personnel. König attended a lecture by Wolf-Dietrich Grodzicki in 1967 at Hamburg University, where the lecturer spoke of a commercial representative who warded off a depression by hypomanic defenses. This was necessary for his work, otherwise the underlying depression would have risen to the surface, with probable loss of contracts with firms with whom he worked. Whether in such a situation the depression could have been healed was doubtful. The speaker decided not to address the hypomanic maneuver, though this had some disadvantageous effects on the patient. A similar situation often faces the psychoanalyst when he works with the chronically ill and with medical personnel. That a psychoanalyst must frame indications and that he has to decide whether the side effects of a therapy are not worse than the illness holds quite generally. Limiting the finding and conveying of truth is a particularly important task with the chronically and fatally ill, as well as with medical personnel.

Chapter 22

The Therapist's Concept of Man

In a therapeutic group the therapist observes each patient interacting with the leader and the other patients. The basis of observation is thus wider than in individual analysis. However, the samples of behavior observed are not in all respects representative of daily life.

Because in groups regression appears and can be reversed more quickly than in individual analysis, the group psychotherapist can more readily observe various stages of rising and receding regression. He will thus tend not to see his patients as children but keep in view their more adult sides, which are presented repeatedly, so that in the end he will gain a more accurate picture of their social skills than will the individual therapist. The therapist's behavior in the group, indeed, even his perception, is influenced by the theoretical concepts he uses.

How can human pictures formed by group therapists using multipersonal concepts be distinguished from those formed by therapists who use dyadic concepts? In the former case, the therapist seems more interested in the behavior of people in varied social relations. His concept of man is of a *homo politicus*. A therapist using unifying concepts is more focused on group fantasies and his concept is one of *homo ludens* (Huizinga 1987), who plays in his fantasy.

An analyst who uses a dyadic concept knows, of course, that the social side matters, and one who uses sociopsychological concepts knows that fantasy matters, but their emphases differ.

A therapist who more often takes up the shared fantasies and less the manifold multipersonal relations will point the patients' attention to what they share, in particular their joint fantasies. A therapist who gives more attention to multipersonal relations will direct the patients' attention to their mutual relations, which gives more weight to behavior as compared with fantasizing. In thus applying his concepts in therapeutic action, the therapist changes the field of observation in a way that corresponds to his interests and brings it nearer his concept of man.

A therapist's concept of man expresses itself in the aims of his treatment. Quite generally, every psychotherapist aims to make his patients better and healthier. What, however, *is* a healthy person? A therapist who values active fantasy will emphasize creativity and regard his patients' everyday social skills as less important. He will also give more rein to his patients in applying their fantasies in daily life than would a therapist who uses a sociopsychological concept. The latter will keep this application in view and promote the transfer from group to daily life by perhaps encouraging patients to report on their experiences outside the group. His groups will be less at risk of becoming a club of emotions (Battegay 1979). Conversely, he may run the risk of neglecting the importance of fantasy and its therapeutic effects, and to dismiss it too soon as to its ability to be put to some use.

Part of a concept of man is the notion of health. If we ask what the term *health* means, we must also ask what *normal* means. The two concepts cannot be severed. One can start from statistical or ideal normalcy. The latter will depend strongly on one's own subjective outlook.

More than in Freud's time, people today must cope with their inner tensions arising from manifold identifications that occur because social roles change so quickly. For example, the notion of a woman's role in work and at home differs markedly between generations (see Brocher 1967).

Identification with persons of the primary family runs into conflict with role expectations and offers from peers. Today a woman therapist will rarely have had a mother in a profession who was an example of how to combine and harmonize the roles of professional, housewife, and mother. For men, too, it is a problem to adapt to a woman who does not live as they were used to from their own mothers. The varying role identities react on the ideal concept that a therapist can have of how people should be.

As patients in a group we would hope that our therapist has a broader view of what may be regarded as normal or average. He should not see the ideal in a fixed image, but should have different pictures of people who correspond to the various possible environments, tendencies, gifts, and life forms. The more a psychotherapist has to deal with different types of people, in age and social class, the more varied his notion of normalcy. We should welcome it if he had gathered wide social experience and would continue to do so. However, we should likewise hope that he would not regard illness and suffering as normal and to be accepted. He should not draw the line between neurotic suffering and unavoidable ordinary grief in such a way that much of what is therapeutically treatable belongs to the latter kind (see Lindner 1981, 1982). A group psychotherapist has to frame indications. No therapist can entirely eliminate personal sympathies entering an indication. Indeed, they play an important role (see, e.g., Rudolf et al. 1988). However, as experience grows, the spectrum of patients a psychotherapist can work with will grow.

The question of whether we can help a patient contains the question of whether he can work with us. This is among other things a question of skills: Is the patient able to work in a group? Some therapists lose sight of the fact that a patient in a group must do a qualified form of work. What kind of work depends on the therapist's theoretical concepts and his concepts of man. Both influence his concrete work experience with his patients. If he sees a patient more as *homo ludens*, he should not forget that one reason for playing is to gain skills. A child, after all, also learns by playing.

Transforming what has been learned into social skill is a process of trial and error. Insight does not in some magic manner create social skill. A working process mediates between playing in fantasy, the insight so gained, and skillful interpersonal dealings. Conversely, it is peculiar to analytic psychotherapy in groups that it distinguishes between procedures, learning, the playing in fantasy and interaction in the group, on the one hand, and optimizing daily life, on the other. Both are important and should be correlated.

References

Ahrens, S. (1987). Alexithymie und kein Ende? Versuch eines Resümees. *Zeitschrift für Psychosomatische Medizin und Psychoanalyse* 33:201–220.

Argelander, H. (1972). *Gruppenprozesse: Wege zur Anwendung der Psychoanalyse in Behandlung, Lehre und Forschung.* Reinbek: Rowohlt.

_____ (1979). *Die kognitive Organisation psychischen Geschehens.* Stuttgart: Klett-Cotta.

Battegay, R. (1975). Defective developments of therapeutic groups. In *Gruppentherapie und soziale Umwelt*, ed. A. Uchtenhagen, R. Battegay, and A. Friedman, pp. 373–374. Bern/Stuttgart/Wien: Huber.

_____ (1979). *Der Mensch in der Gruppe.* Bern: Huber.

Bellak, L., Hurvich, M., and Gediman, H. K. (1973). *Ego Functions in Schizophrenics, Neurotics and Normals.* New York: Wiley.

Bion, W. R. (1961). *Experiences in Groups and Other Papers.* London: Tavistock.

Bischof, N. (1985). *Das Rätsel Ödipus.* München: Piper.

Biskup, J. (1991). *Die Verarbeitung chronischer Krankheit unter psychoanalytischem Aspekt*. Göttingen: Examensarbeit am Institut für Psychotherapie und Psychoanalyse.

Blanck, R. and Blanck, G. (1974). *Ego Psychology: Theory and Practice*. New York/London: Columbia University Press.

Brocher, T. (1967). *Gruppendynamik und Erwachsenenbildung*. Braunschweig: Georg Westermann.

Cohn, R. (1984). Themenzentrierte Interaktion. Ein Ansatz zum Sich-selbst-und Gruppenleiten. In *Die Psychologie des 20. Jahrhunderts, Bd. 2: Sozialpsychologie*, ed. A. Heigl-Evers and U. Streeck, pp. 873–883. Weinheim/Basel: Beltz.

Davies-Osterkamp, S., Heigl-Evers, A., Bosse-Steuernagel, G., and Alberti, L. (1987). Zur Interventionstechnik in der psychoanalytisch-interaktionellen und tiefenpsychologisch fundierten Gruppentherapie — eine empirische Untersuchung. *Gruppenpsychotherapie und Gruppendynamik* 23:22–35.

Durkin, H. (1965). *The Group in Depth*. New York: International Universities Press.

Eissler, K. R. (1953). The effect of the structure of the ego on psychoanalytic technique. *Journal of the American Psychoanalytic Association* 1:104–143.

Erdheim, M. (1988). *Die Psychoanalyse und das Unbewusste*. Frankfurt: Suhrkamp.

Ermann, M. (1985). Die Fixierung in der frühen Triangulierung. *Forum der Psychoanalyse* 1:93–110.

Ezriel, H. (1960/1961). Übertragung und psychoanalytische Deutung in der Einzel–und Gruppenpsychotherapie. *Psyche* 14:496–523.

Faber, F. R. and Haarstrick, R. (1989). *Kommentar Psychotherapie-Richtlinien*. München: Jungjohann Verlagsgesellschaft.

Foulkes, S. H. (1977). *Therapeutic Group Analysis*. 2nd ed. New York: International Universities Press.

—— (1990a). Group-analytic psychotherapy. Text and three tapes dictated by the author. Joint Publications Committee of the Institute of Group Analysis and the Group-Analytic Society, London.

—— (1990b). *Selected Papers: Psychoanalysis and Group Analysis*. London: Karnac Books.

Frank, K. (1986). Die Abstinenz und die Freiheit des Analytikers. *Gruppenpsychotherapie und Gruppendynamik* 21:181–193.

Freud, S. (1904). Freud's psycho-analytical procedure. *Standard Edition* 7:249–256.

_____ (1912). Papers on technique: recommendations to physicians practicing psycho-analysis. *Standard Edition* 12:109–120.

_____ (1914). Papers on technique: remembering, repeating and working-through. *Standard Edition* 12:145–156.

_____ (1927). The future of an illusion. *Standard Edition* 21:3–58.

_____ (1928). New introductory lectures on psycho-analysis. *Standard Edition* 22:3–6.

_____ (1937a). Analysis terminable and interminable. *Standard Edition* 23:209–215.

_____ (1937b). Constructions in analysis. *Standard Edition* 23:255–270.

Fürstenau, P. (1979). *Zur Theorie psychoanalytischer Praxis: Psychoanalytisch-sozialwissenschaftliche Studien*. Stuttgart: Klett-Cotta.

Garland, C. (1982). Group analysis: taking the non-problem seriously. *Group Analysis* 15:4–14.

Gill, M. M. (1954). Psychoanalysis and exploratory psychotherapy. Journal of the American Psychoanalytic Association 2:771–797.

Glover, E. (1955). *The Technique of Psychoanalysis*. London: Ballière, Tindall & Cox.

Greenson, R. R. (1967). *The Technique and Practice of Psychoanalysis*. New York: International Universities Press.

Grotjahn, M. (1979). *Analytische Gruppentherapie: Kunst und Technik*. München: Kindler.

_____ (1983). Group communication and group therapy with the aged. In *Handbook of Group Psychotherapy*, ed. M. Grotjahn, F. M. Kline and C. Friedmann, pp. 149–154. New York: Van Nostrand Reinhold.

Heigl, F. (1969). Zum strukturellen Denken in der Psychoanalyse. In *Aspekte der Psychoanalyse*, ed. A. Schelkopf and S. Elhardt, pp. 12–25. Göttingen: Vandenhoeck & Ruprecht.

_____ (1987). *Indikation und Prognose in Psychoanalyse und Psychotherapie*, 3rd ed. Göttingen: Vandenhoeck & Ruprecht.

Heigl, F., and Triebel, A. (1977). *Lernvorgänge in psychoanalytischer Therapie*. Bern/Stuttgart/Wien: Huber.

Heigl-Evers, A. (1978). Konzepte der analytischen Gruppentherapie. Göttingen: Vandenhoeck & Ruprecht.

Heigl-Evers, A., and Heigl, F. (1968). Analytische Einzel- und Gruppenpsychotherapie. *Gruppenpsychotherapie und Gruppendynamik* 2:21–52.

_____ (1973). Gruppentherapie: interaktionell–tiefenpsychologisch fundiert (analytisch orientiert)–psychoanalytisch. *Gruppenpsychotherapie und Gruppendynamik* 7:132–157.

────── (1977). Zum Konzept der unbewussten Phantasie in der psychoanalytischen Gruppentherapie des Göttinger Modells. *Gruppenpsychotherapie und Gruppendynamik* 11:6–22.

────── (1979). Die psychosozialen Kompromissbildungen als Umschaltstellen innerseelischer und zwischenmenschlicher Beziehungen. *Gruppenpsychotherapie und Gruppendynamik* 14:310–325.

────── (1983). Das interaktionelle Prinzip in der Einzel – und Gruppenpsychotherapie. Zeitschrift für *Psychosomatische Medizin und Psychoanalyse* 29:1–14.

Heigl-Evers, A., and Hering, A. (1970). Die Spiegelung einer Patientengruppe durch eine Therapeuten-Kontrollgruppe: Darstellung eines gruppendynamischen Prozesses. *Gruppenpsychotherapie und Gruppendynamik* 4:179–190.

Heigl-Evers, A., and Schulte-Herbrüggen, O. W. (1977). Zur normativen Verhaltensregulierung in Gruppen. *Gruppenpsychotherapie und Gruppendynamik* 12:226–241.

Heigl-Evers, A., and Streeck, U. (1985). Psychoanalytisch-interaktionelle Therapie. *Medizinische Psychologie* 35:176–182.

Herdieckerhoff, G. (1989). Funktionen nonverbaler Kommunikation. *Gruppenpsychotherapie und Gruppendynamik* 25:243–251.

Hofstätter, P. R. (1971). *Gruppendynamik*. Reinbek: Rowohlt.

Huizinga, J. (1987). *Homo Ludens: Vom Ursprung der Kultur im Spiel*. Reinbek: Rowohlt.

Jacobson, E. (1964): The Self and the Object World. New York: International Universities Press.

Kadis, A. L., Krasner, J. D., Winick, C., and Foulkes, S. H. (1963). *A Practicum of Group Psychotherapy*. New York/Evanston/London: Harper & Row.

Kendon, A. (1977). *Studies in the Behavior of Social Interaction*. Bloomington, IN: University of Indiana Press.

Kernberg, O. F. (1975). *Borderline Conditions and Pathological Narcissism*. New York: Jason Aronson.

Kernberg, O. F., Selzer, M. A., Koenigsberg, H. W., Carr, A. C., and Apfelbaum, A. H. (1989). *Psychodynamic Psychotherapy of Borderline Patients*. New York: Basic Books.

Koch, T. (1989). *Mit Gott leben*. Tübingen: Mohr.

König, K. (1973). Theoretisches Konzept und Interventionstechnik des Gruppentherapeuten unter Berücksichtigung seiner gruppendynamischen Position. *Gruppenpsychotherapie und Gruppendynamik* 7:158–179.

_____ (1974a). Die Risikobereitschaft des Patienten als prognostisches Kriterium. *Zeitschrift für Psychosomatische Medizin und Psychoanalyse* 21:165–178.

_____ (1974b). Arbeitsbezeihung in der Gruppenpsychotherapie – Konzept und Technik. *Gruppenpsychotherapie und Gruppendynamik* 8:152–166.

_____ (1974c). Induzierte szenische Spontandarstellung (ISS) in therapeutischen Gruppen. *Gruppenpsychotherapie und Gruppendynamik* 8: 15–21.

_____ (1974d). Analytische Gruppenpsychotherapie in einer Klinik. *Gruppenpsychotherapie und Gruppendynamik* 8: 260–279.

_____ (1975b). Der Gebrauch von Rekonstruktionen in der analytischen Gruppe. *Gruppenpsychotherapie und Gruppendynamik* 9: 26–31.

_____ (1975c). Der schweigende schizoide Patient in der analytischen Gruppe. *Gruppenpsychotherapie und Gruppendynamik* 9:185–190.

_____ (1976). Übertragungsauslöser – Übertragung – Regression in der analytischen Gruppe. *Gruppenpsychotherapie und Gruppendynamik* 10:220–232.

_____ (1977). Der Therapeut als Beobachter, Interpret, Schrittmacher und Teilnehmer der Gruppe. *Praxis der Psychotherapie* 12:249–255.

_____ (1979). Gruppentherapie. In *Die Psychologie des 20. Jahrhunderts*, ed. P. Hahn, pp. 900–910. Zürich: Kindler.

_____ (1982). Der interaktionelle Anteil der Übertragung in einzelanalyse und analytischer Gruppenpsychotherapie. *Gruppenpsychotherapie und Gruppendynamik* 18:76–83.

_____ (1984). Unbewusste Manipulation in der Psychotherapie im Alltag. *Georgia Augusta* 40:10–16.

_____ (1985). Basic assumption groups and working groups revisited. In *Bion and Group Psychotherapy*, ed. M. Pines, pp. 151–156. London/Boston/Melbourne/Henley: Routledge & Kegan Paul.

_____ (1986a). Schweigen und Sprechen in psychoanalytischen Gruppen. *Gruppenpsychotherapie und Gruppendynamik* 22:9–21.

_____ (1986b). *Angst und Persönlichkeit: Das Konzept vom steuernden Objekt und seine Anwendungen.* Göttingen: Vandenhoeck & Ruprecht.

_____ (1989). Das Menschenbild in der Gruppenpsychotherapie. *Gruppenpsychotherapie und Gruppendynamik* 25:22–27.

_____ (1990). Zur Vorbereitung und Einleitung einer analytischen Gruppenpsychotherapie. *Gruppenpsychotherapie und Gruppendynamik* 26:101–122.

_____ (1991a). Zur Entwicklung der psychoanalytischen Gruppentherapie.

Praxis der *Psychotherapie und Psychosomatik* 36:24–31.

—— (1991b). *Praxis der psychoanalytischen Therapie.* Göttingen: Vandenhoeck & Ruprecht.

—— (1991c). Group-analytic interpretations: individual and group, descriptive and metaphoric. *Group Analysis* 12:111–115.

—— (1994). Indikation. Entscheidungen vor und wahrend einer psychoanalytischen Therapie. Göttingen: Vandenhoeck & Ruprecht.

König, K., and Kreische, R. (1991). *Psychotherapeuten und Paare.* Göttingen: Vandenhoeck & Ruprecht.

König, K., and Sachsse, U. (1981). Die zeitliche Limitierung in der klinischen Psychotherapie. In *Psychotherapie im Krankenhause,* ed. F. Heigl and H. Neun, pp. 168–172. Göttingen: Vandenhoeck & Ruprecht.

Kreische, R. (1986). Die Behandlung von neurotischen Paarkonflikten mit paralleler analytischer Gruppentherapie für beide Partner. *Gruppenpsychotherapie und Gruppendynamik* 21:337–349.

Kris, E. (1936). *Psychoanalytic Explorations in Art.* New York: International Universities Press.

Kutter, P. (1971). Übertragung und Prozess in der psychoanalytischen Gruppentherapie. *Psyche* 25:856–873.

Lichtenberg, J. D. (1983). *Psychoanalysis and Infant Research.* Hillsdale, NJ: Analytic Press.

Lindner, W. -V. (1976). Zur Konzeption der analytischen Gruppentherapie. *Wirklichkeit und Wahrheit* 2:74–83.

—— (1981). Existentieller und neurotischer Konflikt. In *Der Krankheitsbegriff in der Psychoanalyse,* ed. H. Bach, pp. 36–46. Vandenhoeck & Ruprecht.

—— (1982). Existentielle und neurotische Angst. *Praxis der Psychotherapie und Psychosomatik* 27:33–40.

—— (1987a). Überlegungen aus der Sicht des Praktikers. *Gruppenpsychotherapie und Gruppendynamik* 23:19–21.

—— (1987b). Psychoanalytisch orientierte Suchtkrankentherapie. In *Psychiatrie-Plenum,* ed. R. Koechel and D. Ohlemeier, pp. 65–72. Berlin/Heidelberg/New York: Springer.

—— (1988). Von der Inszenierung innerseelischer Konflikte in der Gruppe. In *Gruppenanalytische Exkurse,* ed. D. V. Ritter-Röhr, pp. 71–77. Berlin/Heidelberg/New York: Springer.

—— (1989). Indikation und Ziele in der analytischen Gruppenpsychotherapie. *Gruppenpsychotherapie und Gruppendynamik* 25:35–39.

—— (1990a). Die Beendigung einer psychoanalytisch geführten Gruppe.

Gruppenpsychotherapie und Gruppendynamik 26:123–144.

———— (1990b). Begegnung mit Fremden. *Praxis der Kinderpsychologie und Kinderpsychiatrie* 39:210–214.

———— (1991a). Was hat sich gewandelt in der Gruppenpsychotherapie? In *Psychotherapie im Wandel — Abhängigkeit.* ed. P. Buchheim, M. Cierpka, and T. Seifert, pp. 100–112. Berlin/Heidelberg/New York: Springer.

———— (1991b). Trennung, Abschied und Trauer. In *Suchttherapie — psychoanalytisch, verhaltenstherapeutisch,* ed. A. Heigl-Evers, I. Helas, and C. Vollmer, pp. 181–189. Göttingen: Vandenhoeck & Ruprecht.

Luborsky, L., Mintz, J., Auerbach, A. et al. (1980). Predicting the outcomes of psychotherapy: findings of the Penn psychotherapy project. *Archives of General Psychiatry* 37:471–481.

Mahl, G. F. (1970). *Expressive behavior during the analytic process.* Unpublished manuscript, Yale University.

Mahler, M. S. (1968). *On Human Symbiosis and the Vicissitudes of Individuation.* Vol. I: *Infantile Psychosis.* New York: International Universities Press.

Malan, D. H. (1976). *Toward the Validation of Dynamic Psychotherapy.* New York: Plenum.

Menninger, K. A., and Holzman, P. S. (1958). *Theory of Psychoanalytic Technique.* New York: Basic Books.

Mentzos, S. (1976). *Interpersonale und institutionalisierte Abwehr.* Frankfurt: Suhrkamp.

Ogden, T. H. (1979). On projective identification. *International Journal of Psycho-Analysis* 60:357–373.

———— (1982). *Projective Identification and Psychotherapeutic Technique.* Northvale, NJ: Jason Aronson.

Ohlmeier, D. (1975). Gruppenpsychotherapie und psychoanalytische Theorie. In *Gruppenpsychotherapie und soziale Umwelt,* ed. A. Uchtenhagen et al., pp. 548–557. Bern: Huber.

———— (1976). Gruppeneigenschaften des psychischen Apparates. In *Die Psychologie des 20. Jahrhunderts. Bd. 2: Tiefenpsychologie,* ed. D. Eicke, pp. 1133–1144. Zurich: Kindler.

Ott, J. (1991). Die psychoanalytisch-interaktionellen Vorgehensweisen in der psychoanalytisch orientierten Gruppentherapie. Vortrag auf den 41. Lindauer Psychotherapiewochen 1991.

Pines, M. (1972). Basic principles, changes and trends. *Group Analysis* 5:85–91.

Racker, H. (1953). Contribution to the problem of countertransference. *International Journal of Psycho-Analysis* 34:313–324.

Rohde-Dachser, C. (1982). Diagnostische und behandlungstechnische Probleme im Bereich der sogenannten Ich-Störungen. *Psychotherapie Psychosomatik Medizinische Psychologie* 32:14.

Rotmann, M. (1978). Über die Bedeutung des Vaters in der "Wiederannäherungsphase." *Psyche* 32:1105–1147.

_____ (1985). Frühe Triangulierung und Vaterbeziehung. *Forum der Psychoanalyse* 1:308–317.

Rudolf, G., Grande, T., and Prosch, U. (1988). Die Berliner Psychotherapiestudie. *Zeitschrift für Psychosomatische Medizin und Psychoanalyse* 34:2–18.

Sandler, J. (1960). The background of safety. *International Journal of Psycho-Analysis* 41:352–356.

_____ (1976). Countertransferences and role-responsiveness. *International Review of Psycho-Analysis* 3:43–47.

Sandner, D. (1990). Modelle der analytischen Gruppenpsychotherapie – Indikation und Kontraindikation. *Gruppenpsychotherapie und Gruppendynamik* 26:87–100.

Scharfenberg, J. (1968). *Sigmund Freud und seine Religionskritik als Herausforderung für den christlichen Glauben.* Göttingen: Vandenhoeck & Ruprecht.

Scheflen, A. E. (1964). The significance of posture in communication systems. *Psychiatry* 27:316–321.

Scheidlinger, S. (1964). Identification, the sense of identity and of belonging in small groups. *International Journal of Group Psychotherapy* 14:291–301.

Schindler, R. (1957/1958). Grundprinzipien der Psychodynamik in der Gruppe. *Psyche* 11:308–314.

Schindler, W. (1951). Family pattern in group formation and therapy. *International Journal of Psychotherapy* 1:100–105.

_____ (1966). The role of the mother in group psychotherapy. *International Journal of Group Psychotherapy* 16:189–200.

Sluzki, C. E., and Ransom, D. C., eds. (1976). *Double Bind: The Foundation of the Communicational Approach to the Family.* New York: Grune & Stratton.

Sterba, R. F. (1934). The fate of the ego in analytic therapy. *International Journal of Psycho-Analysis* 15:117–126.

Stern, D. (1985). *The Interpersonal World of the Infant.* New York: Basic Books.

Stock-Whitaker, D., and Liebermann, A. (1965). *Psychotherapy through the Group Process.* London: Tavistock.

Stolzenberg, E. (1986). *Wann ist eine Psychoanalyse beendet? Vom idealistisch-*

normativen zum systemischen Ansatz. Göttingen: Vandenhoeck & Ruprecht.

Strachey, J. (1934). The nature of the therapeutic action of psychoanalysis. *International Journal of Psycho-Analysis* 15:127-186.

Streeck, U. (1980). "Definition der Situation," soziale Normen und interaktionelle Gruppenpsychotherapie. *Gruppenpsychotherapie und Gruppendynamik* 16:209-221.

Ticho, E. A. (1971). Probleme des Abschlusses der psychoanalytischen Therapie. *Psyche* 25:44-56.

Winnicott, D. W. (1956). Primary maternal preoccupation. In *Through Pediatrics to Psychoanalysis*, pp. 300-305. London: Hogarth Press, 1975.

―― (1958). The capacity to be alone. *International Journal of Psycho-Analysis* 39:416-420.

―― (1974). *The Maturational Processes and the Facilitating Environment.* New York: International Universities Press.

Wolf, A. (1971). Psychoanalyse in Gruppen. In *Psychoanalytische Therapie in Gruppen*, ed. S. de Schill, pp. 145-149. Stuttgart: Klett.

Yalom, I. D. (1974). *The Theory and Practice of Group Psychotherapy.* New York: Basic Books.

The following chapters of this book are based upon earlier publications:

"Introduction" (König 1977)

"Transference Triggers and the Course of Groups" (König 1976)

"Working Relations" (König 1974b, 1977)

"Interventions" (König 1975b, 1974c)

"Behavior of Therapist and Patients Specific to Structure and Transference" (König 1986a)

"Preparation and Initiation of an Analytic Group Psychotherapy" (König 1990)

"On Ending a Group" (Linder 1990a)

"Inpatient Psychotherapy from the Group Perspective" (König 1974d)

"Group Psychotherapy and Group Dynamics" (König 1977)

"The Therapist's Concepts of Man" (König 1989)

Index